DREAM CHASER

HEITH

ISBN 979-889443860-3

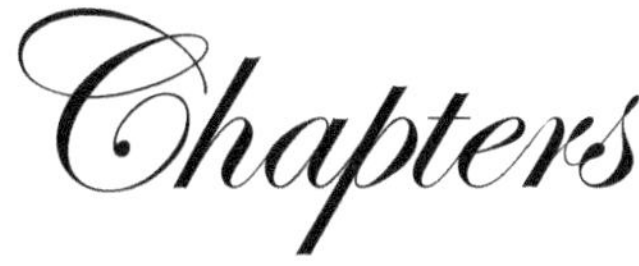

Introduction

The summer of 2022. I swear I don't remember it raining once, although I'm sure it did a couple of times. It was a dry summer and hot. We had a couple months off work for different reasons and spent every day possible embracing what felt like the best summer ever. Trips to this little beach that was located close by became our favorite place to go, absorbing the sun. We knew it was a special time and were blessed to have had it. We sat and I began talking about my life. This is when a recorder was turned on and the typing began.

Who am I, and why should I write a book about myself? So many people have their own stories to tell. Why should I and what's so special about me? Sometimes I feel like I've had a tough life, and then I feel guilty for feeling that way. I think about how many other people have had it much worse. At times I feel like I have no right to complain, but everything in life is relative. That's their story and this is mine, and it's an interesting journey.

Names have been changed to protect everyone.

Chapter 1

In the Beginning

So, I grew up in a neighborhood that was called Silver Lake. Well, we moved there in 76 after leaving Central Falls. Silver Lake wasn't a bad neighborhood, but then again when you're a little kid you don't really see the good or bad much. It just is what it is, everything is relative in life. You can grow up in a place that's a zoo and that just seems normal. You can live a privileged life, and then usually expect life just to be that way.

The first building block in every child's foundation is set by their mother or mother figure. I was very close to my mother when I was a small child. I was a stuttering, anxious mess and attached to her like glue. Like most kids, I thought she was perfect until I got a little older. I guess the first sign of things being not so perfect was the first time she disappeared. I was little and I went to stay with friends of my parents. I later learned, "Moms in the hospital getting better."
My mother's side of the family has a whole history of mental health issues. My grandmother Ann died from driving her car into a telephone pole at the age of forty-nine. It was a residential neighborhood with short narrow streets. There

was no way she was driving fast enough to hit the pole hard enough that it would kill her unless she did it on purpose. From the stories I've heard, suicide seems likely. Oddly enough, I found out that I lived in that same neighborhood for years. I raised my youngest daughter for the first 13 years of her life, on the next street over from where my grandmother had died forty something years earlier.

My mom's dad, my grandfather, died in Vegas, he was affiliated with organized crime. I'm 99% sure he was murdered. He owned a restaurant called the White Shark. I can remember being little and hearing my parents talking softly one night. My mother was saying how there was blood all over the walls. I was young, and to be honest, it was disturbing. I remember saying to her, "What do you mean, whose blood was on the walls? ". After a short pause she said, "Oh your grandfather was sick, and he hemorrhaged ". Meaning like he was throwing up blood because he was sick, but that wasn't the case. I wasn't stupid. From what I heard being said, it was because he was shot or something gruesome happened. I was certain of it.

My mom had three brothers in all, Uncle James, Adam, and Albert, plus a sister Karen. They grew up in South Providence. Uncle James only came around on special occasions. It was always exciting because he was mysterious. I knew he had arrived when I saw the big Cadillac logo on that big shiny chrome grill roll into the driveway. The car seemed huge to me. He was in his 1970's polyester suit and leather jacket. You could see the bulge in his jacket where his gun was tucked in by his waist. My mom would be so excited too. She adored him. He was her big brother and he taught her how to survive.

He was a Gangsta, and my mom was damn proud of it. My

uncle started off with a Wiener Joint where he had fur coats and thousand-dollar suits rolling in and out of the back door. That was before I was born. Fencing was his thing. He later owned a steak house in East Greenwich. An expensive place to eat. As soon as my grandfather "hemorrhage", Uncle James sold the restaurant, and left for Las Vegas. I didn't see him again until I was an adult myself. He lived there in Vegas for the rest of his life.

They grew up poor. My mother needed to search for food to eat when she was a kid. Her big brother James taught her where and how to get what she needed to survive. He was the oldest, and I guess the one everyone looked up to. Back in the 50's there were a lot of food delivery trucks on the road. Delivering things like milk and bread products to homes. My mother wasn't even ten years old when she needed to not only steal food, but her clothing as well. Walk in wearing her rags and walking out with a new outfit for school. not like she made it to school often.

They used to shop lift for clothes, not to have nice clothes. They did it just to have clothes to wear. Poverty was the least of her problems though, the abuse is what destroyed her. She was set up to fail from day one. Her dysfunctional childhood would sure pave the way for her challenging life.

I knew my uncle Albert pretty good. When I was a kid, my mom was close to him. I had two cousins, Anthony and Maria. Somewhere along the way we lost contact. I'm pretty sure my parents borrowed money from him and didn't give it back. It got so ugly I didn't see him again for a very long time. Not until I was an adult and old enough to smoke a joint with him. He was a cool dude. For a while in my early twenties, we got together often to hangout and smoke.

He had tattoos and face piercings. He was down to earth. He had a young girlfriend. Some people were talking shit about him because he wasn't acting his age, whatever that is supposed to mean. Like he wasn't doing anything wrong. Guy was like fifty-five just trying to live his life after battling a life full of shitty shit. Still to this day we talk from time to time.

Growing up, Uncle Adam was the most mysterious uncle I didn't see. All I knew was that he was in prison my entire childhood. He went to jail for robbery. A few of them, I think. He was involved in stuff too. Trying to survive like James who seemed to be a success at it, I guess. He was eventually released, he showed up at my parents one day. I was an adult by then, living on my own. So, I did meet him a few times.

He was an interesting person, very quiet. He was in the Korean war. I believe he suffered from PTSD from it. He fought on the ground. He saw and did a lot, it was war. My mother used to tell me that "he lost it over there". He had a colorful life, and I don't know enough to get into it. I was never given the opportunity to get close to him at all. Ironically, he played a significant role in my existence.

I didn't hear much about Aunt Karen. I know my mother had mixed feelings about her. My grandmother was an alcoholic, and she went out drinking a lot. She would come home late, wake all the kids up out of bed and strip them down naked. She would make my mother, Albert, and Adam, who were the three youngest, kneel on dry uncooked rice as their mother beat their bare skin with a belt. Aunt Karen would assist at times, instead of helping her siblings. The truth is she was probably petrified and was grateful to not be beaten herself. Although she probably was at one time too. The oldest, Uncle James, was out in the streets. Not sure if my mother ever really forgave my aunt. As an adult my aunt had apologized to my mother, I think it was too late at that point, The damage was too deep.

There is no denying that there are some jacked up genetics on my mom's side. Even her closest cousin died from a drug overdose after losing his wife. One day his wife was trying to go out alone for the afternoon, and he gave her a hard time. "Take one of the kids", he kept saying. They argued and she ended up taking their oldest daughter out with her.

Unfortunately, she was heading down to the train tracks. She stood by the rails waiting. As a train approached, she pushed her daughter backwards in the opposite direction as she leaped in front of the moving train herself. The poor kid wasn't even ten years old yet. When the first responders arrived all the little girl could say was, "Mommy is everywhere", repeatedly.

Years later that then little girl was spotted at the bus station dirty, pregnant, covered in homemade tattoos asking for money. We are so vulnerable as humans. Being a parent is such a commitment, and way too many just don't get it. One bad choice and ya kid is traumatized for life.

When you're a kid you hear things, people talking. They don't think that kids hear what they are saying. When I was a kid, I knew that they didn't think I understood, but I more than often did. That led to me hearing some shit that I wish I didn't, to say the least. Some things I remembered and figured out a little later.

My mother, my mother, oh does my heart ache for her.

Before I was born my mother had a liking for Barbiturates, apparently. I knew this because I heard it said so many times when I “wasn’t listening”. Barbiturates, whatever the hell that was anyways, then. To me that meant my mother liked to party, as it sounded. Later in life realized what that meant. She was self-medicating.

She didn’t really drink often that I remember. I think her abusive, alcoholic mother scared her away from alcohol. She would only drink here and there when she was manic. I’m glad it wasn’t a regular thing because she would become difficult when she did drink. It was always too much and mixed with her prescription medications. Whatever condition she was in mentally, became ten thousand times worse. She liked to drink Amaretto with coke on the holidays. The most popular time to drink was Christmas, which would absolutely ruin the day like clockwork.

We would never know when money would be good. My mother’s Manic behavior controlled our financial stability or lack of. We had a beautiful home but sat around the electric stove to keep warm on many cold winter nights, often enough to remember. Somehow, they were generous at Christmas. Although, the best gift would have been a peaceful Christmas.

I have this one photo of my parents sitting in front of the Christmas tree with forced smiles. I was so excited because it was Christmas day. I wanted it to be great, but moments before I took that photo my mother was fighting with my father over God knows what. The camera went flying across the room. I begged them to let me take one nice picture for Christmas.

My mother could be hard at times. She lacked empathy. One Christmas, a while after I had left home my sister and brother bought her gifts from the school Christmas store. She opened the gift from my sister. Everyone could tell that my mother was disappointed with the gift. My mother cruelly said, "This is all you got me with the money you spent?". Apparently, she had begun drinking.

What she said was upsetting. I felt so bad for my little sister. Now my uncle Albert was there. For some reason this mysterious uncle appeared and was at my parents' house for Christmas. He was a struggling alcoholic himself. I walked over to the counter and grabbed the liquor bottle. As I was pouring it out in the sink, my uncle just looked at me. Then he said, "I don't think your mother is going to be happy about that". I told him that I didn't care. Then he said, "I wouldn't blame her if she was mad ". He was nice about it.

Well, she went to pour herself another glass and realized that it was gone. I told her that I dumped it out because she couldn't handle it anymore. To no surprise my uncle was one hundred percent accurate. She was super mad! She charged at me in anger. Jumped at me with a committed leap. She would do that if she was pissed off enough. Hands out, going for the throat. She would have zero self-control at times. It would be a little frightening. She was a small person, but powerful.

She was damaged beyond repair. She would do random things like the time she called Child Protective Services. She said that my then wife and I were drug addicts and neglecting our baby, my son Jr. I was insulted beyond words. At that point I was far from a drug addict. I hadn't even smoked weed yet. For a nineteen-year-old, I was a damn good dad. Child Protective Services came to inspect the house and my son. They Stripped him down; they had checked his body for bruises and stuff. Imagine that? Imagine how humiliated I felt. This happened while I was at work. She would give me things and later say that I stole it. Even calling police on me.

She loved me to death though, as insane as that may sound, go figure. She was a very sick woman, struggling her whole life. She was a damaged person, and she was super lucky when she met my father. He was by her side until the end. There is absolutely nothing she could have done to push him away, nothing! I know this because she did it all to him and he still never left her. He made it possible for her to live as normal of a life as humanly possible when all odds were against her.

My mother had clear cut bipolar, with clear cut symptoms of hopeless suicidal depression and damaging Mania. She also had excessive OCD with cleanliness. Even hallucinating in psychosis. I wasn't allowed to touch the furniture in my own bedroom because the acid in my skin would ruin the finish on the wood. I couldn't cook or make a meal until I left home because I wasn't trusted to clean up after myself thoroughly enough. No water spots could be left behind in the sink or tub. Couldn't walk on the rugs, we had to walk around them. There was a designated brush at the end of a broomstick that we used to cover footprints on the rug if we slipped up and stepped on it. All the fabric in the rug needed to be brushed in the same even direction. It seemed normal, because that's just how it was.

I was very young when I saw my brother Liam fly like superman. When it happened that's exactly what went through my head. My brother just flew from one room into the other like superman flies through the air. From that point on, I didn't defy my mother. I was a bright kid. I did what I was told. I had no interest in flying or being superman.

She suffered from cluster migraine headaches, which understandably made her more irritable. Her neurologist told her it was a result of being hit in the head repeatedly as a child. She was often hit with a high heel shoe. My mother was probably a difficult kid, and her mother wasn't capable of handling her, and raising her or anyone properly.

Mom was always happy to go see the Doctor though. She got her prescriptions. Some meds helped with her headaches. She was great that first week or so. Until she wasn't. Often it would end in her flipping out, accusing everyone of taking her pills. She took a months' worth in about a week. The rest of the month was spent in horror. We were petrified of what she would do and how she would act without her meds, until she got to see the doctor again. Then the cycle would start all over.

This became a way of life for a very long time. Plus, whatever other prescriptions that were also in the mix. As I became older, I realized that the drug addiction she had when she was younger never really went away.

Her survival skills were so strong that she would do whatever it took. She would protect loved ones with the same passion if it did not pose a risk to her own well-being. She was afraid of life. Her fear managed the choices she made every day. That kind of dedication could have gotten her far in life if she was capable of channeling it better. She didn't want to live, but no one would let her die. She did the best she could, even if her best wasn't good enough. It took me years to realize that.

As challenging as things were, I was close to my parents. My Father was everything I wanted to be, when I was a little kid. I remember when I wanted to be just like him. My mother went back to work full-time when I was about eight years old as a Nurse's Aide, as they called it back then. That is when I detached from her and grew to become very close to my father. He worked two jobs; I almost never saw the man sleep. He worked third shift at a Bank in Providence as a HVAC engineer. His office was on the 39th floor. He took me up on the roof of the building one New Year's Eve to watch the fireworks. It was so cool to be looking down at them. It was one of many fond memories with dad.

He worked from midnight to eight in the morning. He came home and took me to school, then went to his second job. I don't remember much time with my mother once she went back to work. She worked fulltime, but also started hanging out with new friends from work. My dad and I spent a lot of time together at that point. One of our favorite things to do was visit this little pond in Scituate where we fed the ducks. We bought bread from the day-old bread store. My father was familiar with this pond before he took me there. I felt like it was an important place to him, and he shared it with me. Since then, I have always enjoyed watching ducks.

My father lost his mother at the age of two. For whatever reasons at the time my grandfather Jose was suspicious of his wife, my father's mother. He had her followed by a private investigator. The discovery was that his suspicions were true. She in fact was cheating on him, with another man. This was 1936 and my grandfather had his wife escorted out by the police. My father was two years old and watched this happen out the kitchen window. My father didn't see his mother again until he was an adult.

There was no question about it. My grandfather instantly had custody of his kids, even though he couldn't really take care of them alone. He worked a lot; it was during the Great Depression. He needed help, so he went to the church. Their recommendation was to give his children up for adoption. He never went to church again after that. He still considered himself religious though, or spiritual. He prayed at home. Alongside his bed he kept a statue of Jesus, Mary, and Joseph, with his bible. It was the same bed that my father was born in during the Great Depression. He kept it his whole life. His home was his church.

Like a lot of kids, my father's grandparents played a big role in raising him. They came from the old country. The first generation in America from the Azores and from Spain. In 1910 they gave birth to my grandfather in America. Growing up without a mother led my father to a life-long struggle, craving a traditional family. He wanted a wife, kids, and a home of his own.

My dad liked to tell me a lot of stories of living back then, "In the old days". They had a bathtub in the basement with shared bath water. The toilet was an outhouse outside in the yard, which was engulfed with fruit trees and vegetables. They weren't dead poor, but during the depression everyone struggled. They were working-class, but poor enough to still not have running water in the house yet. My great grandfather was a tool maker, and then my grandfather also became a tool maker. That's how it was back then. No school was needed, you learned from your father and took on his career. My father was the first in the family to break this, not wanting to be a tool maker himself. By then it also required schooling.

My father was a quiet guy, but he would go against the grain at times if it was important enough to him. In the 50's he was in the military, stationed in Georgia. He was fined for associating with people who were black. He refused to segregate. Segregation was strong and it was an awful time for humanity.

My grandfather was alone, drinking a lot and wasn't doing well mentally. My Dad was so worried that he went AWOL once to check on him. I couldn't tell you what happened, but it was affecting him. One guy took my father's small stature for granted and kept touching his food. My father stuck a fork through his hand. He got in trouble for that, but nobody ever touched his food again.

My Father jumped out of planes in the Airborne. There is when he had an accident that ended his military career early. He went back home to take care of his dad who was alone. His dad's parents had passed by then. He had a daughter who was my father's only sibling, but she was off doing her own thing. My dad was all he had.

He kept his military dress uniform. After all he voluntarily enlisted and wasn't drafted. He wanted to serve his country. This was a decade after World War 2. I still have that uniform hanging in my closet today. It meant so much to him that I've preserved it. Now it means a lot to me too.
My father ended up with one skinny leg; it was because the muscle in that leg was damaged. He struggled with the injury. He had a limp for the rest of his life. He was extremely

self-conscious of his leg and wore long pants almost always, regardless of the temperature. It would have to be damn hot to catch that man in shorts. When he got older, he didn't care as much.

The older ya get, the less you care about what people think of you. It's amazing how much we change mentally as we get older. When we are young, sometimes what others think seems so important to us.

When my dad was younger, he drove nice cars, wore those Sharpe/old school tacky polyester suits. They were in style back then. He lived a bachelor life. A few years later he met Sarah, who he married and had a son with. He bought a house and new car. Worked hard, came home and ate dinner with his family. Just as he had always dreamed. That son was not me. This was before I was born. My father had a family and was living a good life. He wasn't aware that he was the only one that felt that way. He came home from work one day to find divorce papers on the kitchen table waiting for him.

He refused to give her a divorce without a reason, so it went to court. He didn't know why it was happening and he was hurt. She refused to tell him. They hadn't been fighting or anything. He simply didn't understand. He contested the divorce; he didn't want it. He didn't understand why he was losing his family.

In court his then wife said that the main reason for their divorce was because he wanted to play a sex card game together. They were married and this should have been considered a healthy marriage activity. Now mind you this is in the 60s, and it was a different time. He stopped contesting and gave her the divorce. The judge granted it right away. He was humiliated, confused and alone.

Eventually he found out that she was seeing someone else the whole time. Soon after, that new guy moved in with his own kids. My father was doing the weekly visitations with his son. He didn't see his son Toby all week, so he spoiled him on the weekend. Sarah took away everything Toby brought home. She had other kids in the house now and didn't think it was fair that only one kid was given gifts. The others were jealous. She was making it difficult, and he stopped visiting. One thing that upset me about my father was knowing that he stopped seeing his son. His son grew up without him.

I couldn't understand because I always saw him as a nice man because of how he was with my mother, me, and others. I couldn't understand not ever seeing your kid again or even getting up and walking away from your own child, especially a kid. I know the struggle of being a part-time dad. Even good fathers can get a raw deal. Being a father that doesn't live with ya child is difficult.

My dad had some drinking buddies and hung out at the bar. One day a couple of his friends that were brothers introduced my father to their sister. A young pretty girl. He ended up talking to her. They hung out and started dating, they quickly became a couple and moved in together. She became pregnant in that first year. That baby was me.

Chapter 2

God Said Let There Be Light

Seven pounds and eleven ounces, I was born in March of 1972. My mother said that I was planned. She fell in love with my father because she trusted him. They were together for a little over a year when I was born. She told me stories of the day I came into the world. My mother counted all my fingers and toes, she said. I was born with a birth defect that left my feet pointing in towards each other. When I started walking, I needed to wear braces on my legs for a while to fix them. I remember wearing them and how badly the metal bars gorged up the floors. I am so grateful they took care of that when they did. Life could have been way more difficult.

She and my father had gone through some tough times before they met. They both dreamed of a stable family. My dad was a gentle, caring man. She said that his arms resembled two thick loafs of Italian bread. My father had thick arms from lifting weights. She felt safe with him. My mother had PTSD from being abused as a child. She needed a kind man.

I was a quiet kid. I was never into sports. A pencil, some paper, and a box of crayons is all I needed. I also enjoyed creating things with Legos. I rarely played, I liked to use my imagination and create things. I was always different from the other little kids in school. I think history shows that artists are usually not ordinary. If you were to flip through an old family photo album, you would find many pictures of me sitting on the floor drawing, coloring, or making something.

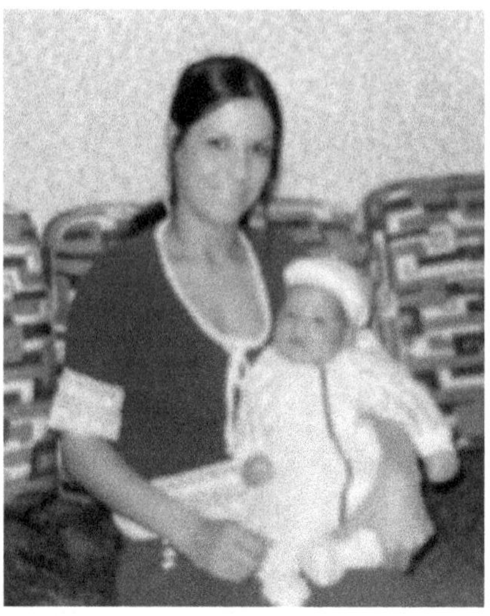

Mom and myself (1972)

I wasn't allowed to use the furniture much, so, I would sit on the floor to draw. When drawing and erasing something, I needed to do it secretly without my mother catching me. I'd try to contain it the best I could and carefully brush the eraser crumbs into the trash. If she saw the crumbs from the eraser, she would become extremely stressed and clean the whole damn room. She had a compulsive disorder with cleaning. I would often be upset because she spent her days off work cleaning the house from top to bottom. She couldn't help it, but it was far from the most significant challenge she had to deal with.

Both of my parents were artistic. My father introduced me to drawing and art itself. My mother could draw well too, but she introduced me to the importance of color. The Art influence at home was strong. Art to me just seemed like something that people did. I assumed everyone was drawing pictures with their families. I didn't know yet that it was something special.

We lived in Pawtucket when I was first born for a few months. The house was run down bad with roaches. My parents didn't want to raise me there, so we moved to an apartment in Central Falls. We lived there until I was four years old. I can close my eyes and describe a walk through that house in detail. Colors of the floors and walls, and room locations. I remember the furniture, pantry and even the yard and neighbors oddly enough.

There was also Sammy, my pet hamster that we kept in a cage behind the stove where it was warm. My mother had two Siamese cats. One of them accidentally scratched my face, leaving a scar. He just missed my eye as he jumped from one chair to another. It was an accident, but I'm pretty sure he was put to sleep. My mother also wanted to get a new cat.

We lived on the third floor in Central falls. The landlord was the chief of police in that city, and his daughter lived on the first floor. One day Liam and I were playing in the yard on the swing, and I don't recall what we did, but we pissed this lady off. Not my mother, but the landlord's daughter. She yelled at us, and we went inside. Shortly after, there was a knock on the door, and it was the lady on the first floor that was just yelling at me a few minutes earlier. This was the police chief's daughter. My mother answered the door, as the lady immediately started yelling at my mother about me and Liam doing something that irritated her.

I can't even remember why; I think we were being too loud maybe. My mother, four feet eleven... maybe. She grabbed this much bigger lady by the hair of her head and brought her down to the floor and beat the shit out of her. She then dragged her by her hair back down to the first floor. Shortly after there was another knock on the door. This time it was the landlord, in full police uniform. I thought my mother was going to jail for sure. Nope, he looked at my mother and said, "what are you doing".

He seemed sympathetic now that I think of it. It was probably obvious that my mother was mentally ill even back then. I hadn't seen it yet. As kids, all we know is what's inside our four walls. That becomes the norm, until we venture out into the world at school age to see how others live.

We moved out of that house shortly after that happened. The truck ride was exciting to me. Everything we owned was in this huge truck. Pulling onto Alverson Ave. I remember it like it was yesterday. Looking at all the houses that were now my new neighbors. The new house had a nice yard.

I experienced being an only child, a little brother, and a big brother. Try to wrap your hands around that math. I have an older brother, there was always some mystery around Liam. My mother gave birth to him when she was sixteen years old. He is seven years older than me but wasn't around at first. I remember a short time prior to Liam being in my world. I can recall the day we picked him up and brought him home with us.

I remember arriving at the house where he was living, and vaguely what the house looked like inside. I was no more than a year old. I clearly recall the day Liam came home and became my big brother. I have this odd ability to remember events when I was extremely young. I can even remember having my diaper changed as a baby.

The story I was told is that Liam was taken away by the state because my mother couldn't take care of him. She was sixteen years old and living together with Liam's father. He was often drunk and hit her. It was when he hit Liam that she left him. It's kind of vague, I don't know exactly what happened. I don't know if she lost Liam due to financial reasons, or her lifestyle. She worked as a dancer; they called them Go-Go girls in the 60s. She danced in cages at clubs. Now that I think about it, maybe it was her mental health that caused Liam to be taken away. Either way she couldn't take care of him and that's why he was in a foster home.

Gotta remember, this was in the 1960s. Things were a lot different than they are now. There were sadly less resources and programs for single abused woman. A lot less understanding. It was a different time. It was before I was born when he went into the foster home. He lived there for the first seven or so years of his life. The sad part is that the foster parents allowed Liam to think that he was their child, as if they were his biological parents. So, I was told.

Liam was getting older and was an energetic child. I'm sure he wasn't treated as well as the foster parent's biological daughter, whom he chased around the yard with a pitchfork one day. That one choice Liam made prompted a call to the state. The foster parents wanted him out. I'm willing to bet by the genetics we all share, he was a handful. I'm also confident that he was only playing and wouldn't have actually hurt their kid with that pitchfork.

Either way the state called my mother who had turned twenty-three. They gave her the option of taking him with her or he would be put up for adoption. She would never have the option of contacting him or seeing him again. She decided that she wanted to welcome him into the family she had just started with my dad. I was recently born earlier that year. My mother and father were building a family together.

Liam was home with me for the first few years of my life. He was my big brother. We were a family. Myself, Liam, and my parents. As Liam got older my mother had a difficult time parenting him. He had a tough start in life and needed special care that my mother probably couldn't provide.

Liam became unpredictable. I heard many conversations as a kid and did my best to put the pieces together in my head. Like one night my mother woke up frightened as he had a sheet over his head, holding a lit birthday cake. Another time he told my mother that he hated my father and me. He wanted our mother and himself to run away and leave my father and me behind. That's when she started to keep a close eye on him. He was caught plotting to scare my dad into a heart attack while he was sleeping, but something happened, and it didn't work out.

Liam had our house searched by detectives with a warrant because he said that my father had stolen merchandise. He didn't... besides some toilet paper and trash bags from work. I remember when the detectives were clearing out our house and packing it into a truck as evidence. They even took our Christmas tree and ornaments, as I cried watching it unfold.

I was told that Liam was caught trying to hurt me as a baby a couple of times. Imagine how many times he maybe didn't get caught doing stuff to me. I feel like maybe he secretly hated me. He was understandably envious I think, but the situation wasn't my fault. I was a toddler, barely walking, when he rolled an old car tire at me. It knocked me down and rolled right over my face. Tires on those cars in the 70s weren't small either.

I also have vague memories of some other compromising situations that aren't so clear. He resented me, and he wanted my mother to himself. I think there was a point that my mother didn't want do deal with him anymore, and he felt it. That sure didn't help. She just didn't know how to handle him. She couldn't provide the special emotional care he probably needed.

He started running away a lot. I'll never forget the day he ran away after setting the kitchen on fire. He was playing with rubbing alcohol and fire for some reason. Police found him a few days later, on the next street over. He was living in a boat in someone's back yard. He didn't go very far. My parents occasionally found ready-to-go run-a-way bags hiding here and there around the house with things like a flashlight, batteries and canned food in it. I remember my father kept saying, "How was he going to eat tuna fish in a can without a can opener". The things you hear as a kid that no one realizes you understand. Many underestimate kids, I don't. Kids are just people in training to become adults from the moment they are born, learning from their surroundings. I was grateful, I thought to myself, at least he put the fire out before he left.

Another time he was missing, and then re-appeared. He claimed that he was kidnapped and taken into a cemetery where some guy had him. There was an actual man that was investigated after being picked up as a suspect. He was picked out in a police lineup. Then my brother came out shortly after and said that it was not true. I'm not sure what happened there. I was too young to fully process it. This is just what I heard. I never doubt what people are capable of. Maybe it was true. I'm sure he was scared. It could have been a lot worse, and I was glad he was ok.

I've heard a lot of things, but I also remember him being nice to me. There was this one time that I was horsing around and broke our mother's cactus. When she came home, she was upset, and Liam took the wrap for it. Maybe he wasn't so bad after all and didn't want to watch me fly like superman too. I'm not sure why he did that, but I did never forget he did that for me. I do have good memories with Liam too.

I believe he was back out of the house before the age of ten years old maybe. I remember visiting him at group homes, and foster homes throughout my childhood. I recall this one place he was in that was so gloomy and it looked like he was in jail to me. It was sad and I recall feeling bad for him. He did come back home and was out again, this went on for a few years. The timeline is a little foggy. I was very young, just going for the ride. The order of some things is a blur. I was a little kid just watching. All I know is that there was a lot of action until Liam was older and was pretty much gone for good. The visits became fewer and further apart. Birthdays and Christmas usually were the only times we saw him.

As I got a little older, I went against my mother's wishes and contacted Liam here and there. We even met up a few times and hung out. Went sledding one winter, that was fun. I still didn't trust him totally, but I also didn't totally trust mom's opinion either. I was becoming an individual with my own mind. Which is probably why I wanted to spend time with him. It was my curiosity that drove me to it, and probably missing out on the feeling of having a brother. My mother drilled into my head never to trust him, and I'm not sure why. I knew we had some situations years back, or maybe there was more to it that was kept from me.

My father was not Liam's biological father, but I was my father's second son. I was the only one he raised though, or even knew to be fair. I learned about Toby, my father's first son when I was about five or six years old. It all happened very fast. He was introduced into the picture somehow spontaneously. Toby grew up being told his father was dead. Once he learned that he was alive, he began to search for him. Toby was nineteen and soon after, he was living with us. Why, I don't know. It was a confusing time, and not much was said to me at that age. I went for the ride.

My parents never went anywhere without me, but this one-night Elvis was performing in Providence. My dad bought tickets. This was just a few weeks before Elvis died. I was usually always with my mother or father; I was still little. They tried to leave me with babysitters in the past a couple of times, but it didn't work out. I would stand somewhere silent for hours, just waiting for them to return. I was troubled but it wasn't noticed yet. But that night, I was left alone with Toby and Liam. I was used to Liam, so I didn't mind so much.

I was in my bedroom, and I heard Toby calling me. I went to see why. Toby was in the bathroom, and he was sitting in the bathtub, naked. The bathroom door was wide open. He was giggling. He had a facecloth covering his penis. I ran back out of the bathroom. I remember being confused. He called me back in again and repeatedly called my name a few times because I hesitated to respond. I slowly walked back into the bathroom, and he pulled the facecloth off himself. I had never seen a grown man naked before, not even my own father.

It was shocking. I was a little kid. I just remember it looking big and hairy. I ran back out, and then Liam appeared in the kitchen, which the bathroom ran off. He was giggling too. The rest is a blur, I can't remember anything else that happened that night. I don't remember Toby leaving the tub, or anything else. I have a great long-term memory, but I cannot remember what happened next. I guess some things are better off not remembered.

The next day Toby was missing. So was the rent money, and even my personal piggy bank that was filled with half dollars. My father used to save them for me when he came across one. Toby didn't come back, and we didn't see him anymore. I never told my parents about what happened. I remember being confused and just afraid to even bring it up. I was little, but I knew it was not ok. Also, all I truly remember was up to seeing him naked and giggling.

Shortly after my father was reading the newspaper to my mother, which he did every day, and became very upset. People seemed to say a lot in front of me thinking I didn't understand, but I did. Toby had been arrested for exposing himself to a child. I don't know anything else about it. I know that my dad was disgusted though. I never told him that he did that to me too. There were a few compromising situations that are halfway burnt into my memory with unclear flashbacks. Not something I like to talk about, but it definitely became a traumatic event in my life.
I've learned to live with flashback and treat them as simple visual memories, good or bad. I hope that blackouts never

clear. I'd rather make believe nothing happened at all. All part of my fight to live a normal life. To not give in to the uglies around me. I haven't seen Toby as an adult. I heard he had a daughter years ago that would be grown by now. I hope he was good to her. I am not sure how I would handle an encounter with him now as a grown man.

Chapter 3

Uncovering My Artistic Skills

I was in kindergarten. The first time I realized that I could draw well. It was my first time in the outside world without my parents. I remember it very well. Day one I had a crush on a girl in my class. Her name was Chrissy, and she had long blond hair. We shared a cubby in the classroom and sat together all day. It was art time, I was excited. The teacher filled the room with easels. We were all told to paint pictures of our family. Chrissy and I had our easels together. So, I painted my house in the background. Mom, dad, myself, even Tommy my cat. It was fun.

The teacher was walking around looking at everyone's work. The usual, telling everyone that they were doing a nice job. When she got to my easel, she paused and didn't say much. She called over two other teachers. Then they all began to praise me. I realized that they were getting really excited about the painting I had made. I wasn't quite sure why, but the feeling of doing something well felt really good. Apparently, it was advanced for a five-year-old in kindergarten.

I was sent home with a letter for my parents to read, recommending they sign me up for art classes. Each year, each new teacher would send home a letter praising my artwork with suggestions to help me expand on it. They scraped the money up and I eventually attended workshops at Rhode Island School of Design a few years later. My father brought me every Saturday for a few years.

I loved the nature room. They had a huge room full of taxidermized animals. I mean every insect to sea creature, birds, bears, tigers and more than anyone could ever imagine. It was amazing. What an opportunity, having any animal you want in front of you to draw. I also learned the fundamentals of drawing a human face and body. I learned a lot there.

I enjoyed making sculptures too. I didn't know they were sculptures when I made them though. I just created stuff all the time. I used cut-up cardboard boxes, duct tape and spray paint. I added miscellaneous functioning things like lights and other components. I just loved to create things that didn't exist already. My father was always impressed with the things I made.

He was my inspiration and biggest fan. **Dad always told me to never give up and to always follow my dreams**. That one piece of advice stuck with me strongly. He taught me how to be a man. How to be a provider. He encouraged art. He was also an artist himself, but he didn't do anything with it, and regretted that.

When in the military he had painted a sign that was a picture of the unit's Mascot. That painting was the first thing that inspired me to become an artist. At that point I became more aware of art and the fact that I liked it and that I was good at it. I started to focus more on it. The idea of becoming an artist became more realistic to me.

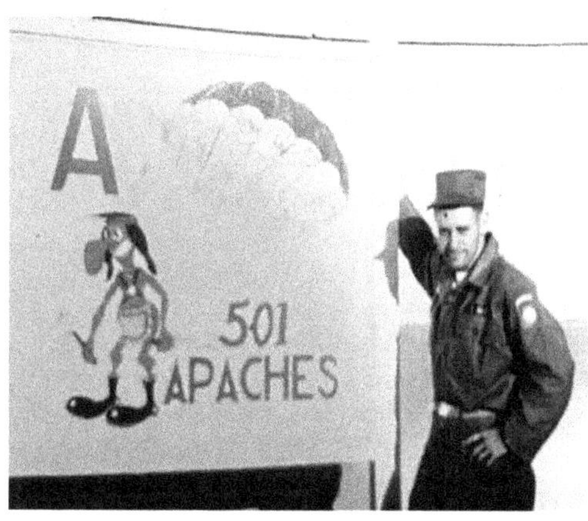

Dad's painting when in the Airborne (1956)

It became obvious at a very young age that art was my talent. When we drove around, I enjoyed looking at the architecture of the buildings. I took notice to the different way each business displayed their business sign. Logos and designs all drew my attention. I noticed aesthetics when most kids my age didn't.

The first time I sold artwork I was in 5th grade. I would almost always be drawing something, every chance I had. I was good at it. People would ask me to draw them cartoons or their name in graffiti. Someone offered me their lunch money once, and I took it. This caught on and I started selling drawings in school every day, in a Catholic school. I'd make five to twenty bucks a day. I got into a lot of trouble with that one. I stayed back because I never did my schoolwork. I just drew pictures every day. I spent a lot of time after school too, cleaning desks as a punishment for drawing all over them during class. Art was all I wanted to do.

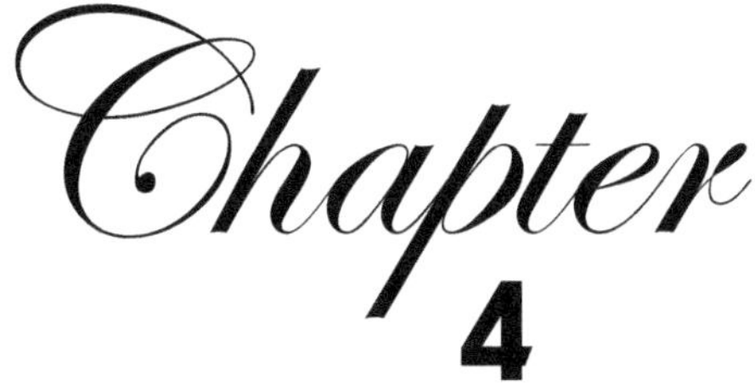

As Far Back as I Can Remember

I was sent to summer day camp during school vacation. While all the kids were playing and participating in a structured outdoor setting. I stood on the side of the field, by the trees watching and waiting. It felt like it would never end. I didn't eat, I just peed my pants standing there. I stood there like a psycho until it was time to go home. Needless to say, I never went back to camp after that day. I was socially petrified. I obviously was not ok.

There was definitely something going on with me. I knew I wasn't like everyone else. When I went to bed at night I needed to pray to God at a very young age. I wanted to, but also, I needed to or else. Which is a good thing, but not how I was. While I prayed, I prayed for everyone in my life individually by name. I asked for them to survive the night. I believed that if I didn't do that there was a 50/50 chance of them not being alive in the morning when I woke up, and it would have been my fault. I believed that without my personal communication with God, there would be havoc and turmoil.

Praying wasn't an easy task as it should have been. For example, I used to recite the "Our father". Seeing and feeling each sentence in the prayer slowly. If I didn't feel that I fully comprehended each word or sentence visually in my mind, it wouldn't be good enough. I would continue and finish, but I would need to do it all over again, and again until I felt that I did it properly. Good enough that God would take me seriously and know that I was sincere. Sometimes it would be once, more than often a few times, but sometimes it could be excessive.

I would see the prayer play out in my head like a video, the entire thing... slide by slide. It was meditation. I would bring my mind all the way to heaven and bring it all the way down to earth but see it in my head. I would visualize flowers rolling out from the sky and spreading across the earth as I imagined, "on earth as it is in Heaven.

I'd be so scared that if I didn't do this, then the house would catch on fire or something bad would happen. People I loved would suffer or die. I had to do this. It was my responsibility to communicate with God and prove that I loved him enough and understood each word of the prayers so he wouldn't take my family away from me. I was done with the prayers when I was satisfied that I understood every word I recited clearly, so God would help me.

Our church as a kid was on the next street from our house, in walking distance. When I was into bikes, that parking lot was the best. There was this one spot where the concrete conveniently created somewhat of a little ramp. Great for little jumps with my bike.

I went to church with my father every Sunday and I started

private school in 3rd grade. They wanted me to have a good education and build solid morals. To be honest, I am grateful for that. With all the challenges, environments and experiences I had ahead of me, that Private school education saved me. It kept that voice in my head reminding me what was right and what was wrong. I would have been an easier target for failure otherwise.

There was a point in my life that I pondered the idea of becoming a priest. That went through my mind briefly. Obviously, this is before I discovered girls. I knew I wasn't an average kid. I wasn't sure what that meant exactly, but I was on a mission to figure it out though.

There are some things that most are not capable of understanding. God asked us to have faith. Doing the right thing is basically what it comes down to. Being positive is important. Creating the right environment for the life you want to live. Treating others as you want to be treated yourself. Trying to understand it fully would be like explaining a smart phone to Christopher Columbus. Humans want to understand everything or have proof. Personally, I believe that God is real. It is proven to me every day!

I suffered in silence; mornings were always challenging. I would more than often wake up in agony with stomach pains. It was always tough getting to school or anywhere scheduled. I'd have to go to use the bathroom several times. The stress of being stuck somewhere inconvenient caused more stress and more stomach pains. I would way too often end up needing to use the bathroom in an inconvenient place and time, with urgency. I've soiled my pants on dates, heading to Job interviews, at work, in traffic. Been stuck with nothing but my socks to wipe. Thank God I have both my feet.

It is a fear everywhere I go to this day. I've been to the doctor's countless times. As an adult I even had a colonoscopy that I woke up during. Most indescribable feeling was waking up as they were pulling the camera out. I opened my eyes to see the monitor in front of me as the camera left ... me. Results were that I had IBS, lucky me, stress goes right to my stomach. I've let it own me most of my life. Like anything else, ya get used to it and learn to live with it.

As a little kid I would lay in bed for hours at night thinking, and not being able to sleep. Sometimes I'd wake up in the middle of the night and have trouble falling back to sleep. We used to keep a bottle of Nyquil in the bathroom cabinet. I guess Mom had given it to me at some point and I must have realized that it knocked me out. I knew that I had a damn good sleep when I had it in the past. Mom may have given it to me just to put me to sleep, I don't know. It was a different time and things that are now questionable weren't so wrong back then. I can't say for sure.

I knew that if I woke up in the middle of the night and couldn't sleep, I wouldn't bother my mother. My father would be working the third shift, overnight. I would stumble into the bathroom and scoot myself up onto the toilet seat. Then I would stand up on it and have full access to the medicine cabinet. No childproof caps then. I'd help myself to God knows how much Nyquil. I guzzled it right out of the bottle like it was water. I slept after that; I always did. I never told my parents, or anyone until I was much older. I guess I knew even then that it was questionable.

Even though we didn't go out much, I spent a lot of time in the car. The family car was a 76 Chevy Impala. Boy, I wish I had that car now. It was huge, I used to hang out in it like it was a club house. That's how big it was inside. My father and I drove my mother to work in it every day. The road we took brought us from the city into the country, and then right into the woods. It was a long road, mostly rural. I remember this little preschool on the right and directly after that on the left was a farmhouse that I always loved. The land was not flat. The house was not pretty. There was nothing attractive about it at all other than the fact that it was by a stream, and plenty of space for chickens and ducks to run around.

Ever since I was little, I always felt as though I was going to be rich one day. I would have land with animals as I dreamed of. I always knew that I would one day be successful. At what, I wasn't sure. I also knew that I would have to make it happen though. I am still working that part out.

I knew that I was gonna have to start early. I saw my parents struggle, and I didn't want that to be me one day as well. I was about twelve when me and my friend started looking for work. We couldn't go far so we walked up and down the main roads nearby, going business to business asking if they were hiring. The problem we had was that we were too young.

I wanted to be a Paperboy. Back then there was an afternoon newspaper and Paperboys would deliver them to houses each day after school. Going home from school on the bus I would see bundles of newspapers on corners waiting for the paperboy to pick up. To be a paperboy, I needed to be fourteen, so I had to be patient because I wasn't old enough.

I was searching for ways to make money. School had fundraisers selling wrapping paper and candy bars. I looked at the back of their catalog one day and contacted the company directly. I found out that I could also do that too. I would buy my own stuff and resell it. That money would go towards earning a profit. So, I did it, I ordered merchandise directly from the catalog. The company charged me one price, I sold it for a higher price. I went door to door doing this and was successful. I eventually did get my own paper route when I was old enough. I was always a hustler though. Being broke will do that to a person.

I was always dreaming of a better life. I often laid in bed thinking. Sometimes it was hard falling to sleep or to stay sleeping. When I did, I often had recurring dreams, so many times that they stuck with me through life. One was me walking alone to school every day and arriving at a large green field with a stone path leading to a split that turned the path into two. Each led to two identical schoolhouses. They both were old, red with white trim and a pointed roof holding a school bell.

Each day I would arrive not knowing which schoolhouse was mine. One was correct and the other one housed a witch that would throw me over the cliff, which was conveniently placed behind the two schoolhouses. I would pick the wrong schoolhouse every time and be thrown over the cliff falling to my demise. I always woke up before hitting the ground.

As a kid I had countless dreams that I woke up to pee, but never actually woke up, or left the bed. I also had repeated dreams that I was riding an elephant naked and feeling so free. I felt the urge to go and was able to freely go while riding the elephant. Of course, I always woke up with a wet bed. Ironically, I somehow did have the opportunity to ride an elephant in real life at one point. I was wearing all my clothes though and did not pee on it.

I was a quiet kid. If I wasn't drawing or building something, I was usually with my cat. It wasn't until I was older that I ventured out. The house I lived in for most of my childhood was in the center of a long road. If you walked to one corner, you were in Hartford Projects. If you walked to the opposite corner, you would be in Silver Lake. My house was just a little closer to that end, but it was almost smack in the middle. We lived there for thirteen years. One end was primarily black, and the other end primarily white Italian. I was neither. When I was old enough to roam, I got along with everyone. I had a very diverse group of friends from both ends.

I didn't do everything my friends did. This is where that Catholic School came in handy. As a teenager some friends stole cars, and went for joy rides, later destroying the cars. And that was the white kids. I could never do that to another person. It's a terrible and cruel thing to do to someone. Car insurance wasn't mandatory back then either. So, some of those poor bastards woke up for work to find their car missing with no way to get to work, and no way to replace their car either.

In the late 70s, early 80s racism was bad, not that it's ever been good. I've witness black kids being escorted out of the white end of my neighborhood. I took no part in that other than voicing my opinion that wasn't always favorable. You must be a certain kind of fucked up in the head to think that a person's skin color determines their character. I knew a bunch of kids that I'd later find out had fathers connected with organized crime. That explained a lot.

At home I hung out in the yard with my dad a lot. I enjoyed helping him with his garden during the summer and listening to him tell me stories of growing up. He and I occasionally walked over to Neutaconkanut Hill. There was a big park there. We would watch some baseball games, but I was never into sports. Christmas time was fun because I got to help dad decorate the outside with lights. He spent a lot of time with me. He took me to shows at the Civic Center every year, Wrestling, Monster truck racing and custom car shows. We had fun. I was lucky to have had him.

We never went very far, no trips out of state or anything. We occasionally did some local stuff in the summer as a family too, and I was happy with it. That's all I knew anyways, and it was good enough. In Rhode Island we had countless beaches, and back then we had Rocky Point amusement park. It was less than a half hour drive away. It was Disney Land to me. They had a huge saltwater pool there that filtered water directly from the ocean. The amusement park been closed for a while, but recently renovated into a nice place to go for a walk by the water. It's a much quieter park now. A few old ride skeletons were left up for nostalgia.

When my mother wanted to spend the day by a saltwater beach, we went to Godard Park. When she wanted fresh water, we went to Pulaski Park Lake. It was only a couple times each summer, but it would be an all-day cookout. It was the highlight of the summer. Neither were very far but it was a day trip for us.

I absolutely hated going clothes shopping with her. She liked to pick me out things like a sweater that would guarantee me to get roasted in school. I went to a private school in a poor neighborhood. In 1980, preppy sweaters didn't fit in . We wore uniforms but come picture day my mother made me wear those stupid sweaters. She liked to fantasize that she was wealthy, and little things like that helped her fulfill her fantasy. I looked good to her, and I know she meant well. My dad would be more understanding and buy me the freshest he could afford. He did his best. Name brands were big then, even in the... unwealthy of neighborhoods.

I had some good times with my mother too though. We occasionally laughed and joked around when her moods were up. I'm glad they took a lot of pictures to remember, because the tough times weigh so heavily. I share memories with my mom during the Blizzard of 78. My mother started shoveling a path from the back door to the street. The snow was up to my nose. We walked to the store together. Everyone was walking that day, because there was so much snow everywhere. The trees were slouched over and looked like dinosaurs to me. It was so cool at six years old.

My mother loved Siamese cats. She had them growing up as a child. Oddly she had them as an adult, even though she had a very bad experience as a kid. One would think she'd want to avoid reminders of a horrific moment in her life. She was a little girl about six years old when her mother's boyfriend threw her cat in the oven. She told me this story repeatedly growing up. The cat started meowing and eventually freaking out until the noise came to an abrupt stop. She was obviously traumatized by it, who wouldn't be. It was another horrifying event in her life.

Growing up, Tommy was the family pet; he was a Siamese cat and a significant part of my life. As silly as it may sound. He was more than just a pet. I remember the day we picked him up from the breeder. I was just about four years old. I was so excited and wanted to see our new kitten's mommy. As we pulled up Liam accidentally poked me in the eye horsing around in the back seat of the car. I couldn't see the mommy cat; my eyes were watering. I was upset and crying.

I spent a lot of time alone drawing or coloring, that's all I enjoyed doing. Tommy became my brother when Liam left for the group homes. Every night at bedtime Tommy had this same annoying, but cute ritual. He would take his paw, and tap on the blanket until I lifted it up high enough for him to suspiciously look in. He'd looked around good to make sure the coast was clear. He walked in slowly, creeping down to the end by my feet. Once he was satisfied, he would come back up and stand there for a minute or so. Just his head showing with his body still under the blanket. If I interrupted him and dropped the blanket before he was done. He would start this process all over again. He wouldn't let me sleep unless I allowed this ridiculousness to take place every night.

I had Tommy until I was twenty-one. That cat meant a lot to me. When I left home at 17, he must have been lost without me. My mother ran hot and cold. She let me take him at one point, then she wanted him back, so I regretfully gave him back. Mom was under five feet tall but intimidating for a little lady. There was no arguing with her. Right or wrong my dad would always defend her. If she argued that the trees were blue and the sky was green, he would agree with her.

Shortly after that she said Tommy was sick. She was taking him to the vet, and he was being put to sleep. I went to see him one last time. He was sitting in the sun, giving me slow blinks. I also knew that my mother wanted new cats, but she could have left Tommy with me. It was hard to tell, with my mother sometimes. He was 17 years old, but she might have rushed it. I'd like to think that Tommy was really just sick, and maybe I just couldn't see it. I was young and maybe in denial. I gave him one last stroke across his fur and walked away.

My father took Tommy to be put to sleep. I went for a walk and kept walking and ended up on the front stairs of a beautiful old church. I was a twenty-one-year-old man crying my eyes out because my cat was being put to sleep. I used to draw pictures of him a lot, one of the first things I ever painted that was good, was when I airbrushed his portrait.

I used to tease Tommy a lot when I was a little kid. I knew he was going to get me back later on. That was the fun in it. Always looking over my shoulder because he was gonna get me back at any time, and I deserved it. It was almost like a game that we played. We sort of had a mutual understanding. He never hurt me, but I'd carry a few scratches. He was a great cat, a beautiful Seal Point Siamese. He was my homie growing up. He was my first portrait. Tommy and imagination... they helped block the uglies out around me. Pets are great, a part of the family. You get unconditional love from them. You get a protector, and a friend.

I always loved animals. Although I've always been a city boy, I dreamed of a farm with countless animals. There is something peaceful about being surrounded by nature. Trees, animals... all of nature's innocence and beauty. When I was a kid and we went to visit family or anywhere, I would immediately look for pets. I could care less if there were kids my age. I preferred simply sitting in the corner petting the cat or dog instead.

Chapter 5

The Gravity of my Mother's Mental Illness

I realized the severity of my mother's declining mental health when I saved her life for the first time, at eleven years old. I was looking for her because I hadn't seen her in a little while. I looked through the house. I checked the basement and the yard. I was calling her name out, yelling, "Mom". She just got her driver's license recently before that and traded in dad's 76 Impala for her new Mercury Cougar. I thought that maybe she might have gone for a ride. Then I realized that I could hear the car running in the garage. I was confused at first because the garage door was closed. I opened the garage door, and indeed there she was.

The car was running. All the windows were rolled down, and the music was blasting loud. She had a nice stereo system installed. The fumes from the exhaust were overwhelming. The car looked empty. I walked up closer to it and saw my mother lying there with the seat all the way back. I yelled her name again. I was very confused. I shook her and she didn't move. I quickly realized what she was doing. I pulled her nearly lifeless body out of that Mercury Cougar. Once out of the garage she got some fresh air, and she woke up. That was the first of many frightening moments that I shared with my mother. Things seemed to get worse fast. Maybe it was because I was older and became more aware. Maybe she realized that I was getting older and could not hide things from me anymore, like she could when I was little.

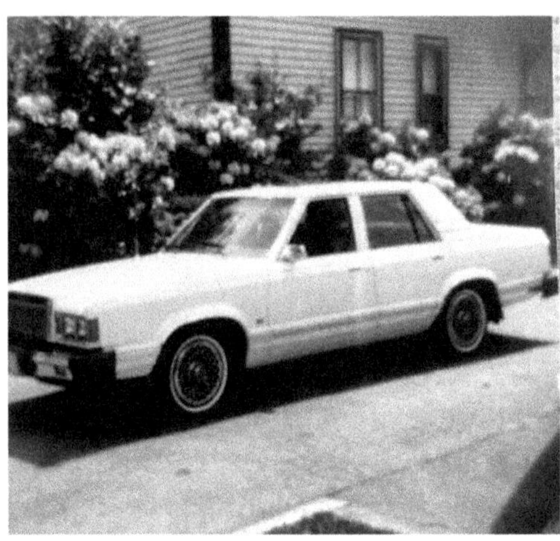

Mom's Mercury Cougar (1983)

The suicide attempts were frightening. At one point I collected every sharp object that I thought she could possibly hurt herself with and hid them well. It was a horrible way to live. I didn't know much difference though. That was how life became.

My mother's depression led to countless suicide attempts. I mean real deal attempts. Rushed to the emergency room kind of stuff. One time I was not home, and she called me mumbling, her voice started to sound like it was fading. She was telling me how much she loved me. It didn't take long before I realized what she had done. My father went to the market, and she swallowed a bunch of pills. I rushed to the house, and of course couldn't get in. I looked through the window and saw her lying limp in bed. I was about to call the police and rescue to break in so I could save her.

I paused for a moment and thought hard about it to myself. I almost didn't make that call. I considered letting her die. Not because I didn't love her, but because I did love her. For a moment, I was going to allow her the chance to finally rest in peace. Then I came to my senses and dialed 911. If I didn't make that call, I would have never forgiven myself.

Going to the hospital became a regular thing. I spent a lot of time visiting my mother in hospitals. I learned how to play pool there from another patient on her unit. This one time she was in the hospital she took the eyeglasses off her own face and literally smashed them on the floor to break them. She took those broken eyeglasses and grinded the shattered glass across her wrist. She wouldn't stop trying to kill herself at all costs. This finally led to her receiving several sessions of electroshock therapy treatments. I was surprised that it was still used for psychiatric treatment. The next day after electroshock therapy she was slow. At first, everything she saw appeared to be as if she was seeing it for the first time ever, including me. It was heartbreaking.

The destruction she had caused herself and to the lives of others around her was overwhelming. I believe that she tried her best. She wasn't equipped with the tools needed mentally. My father was her life support system. She was always in survival mode. Not maliciously to be evil. She was afraid of traumatic history repeating itself.

My father would do anything to make my mother happy. The house we were living in went up for sale. My mother wanted to buy it. The only thing holding them back was a down payment. My father asked his dad for money towards the down payment, and he refused. There was a period of time when there was no communication between my father and grandfather. My father was upset with him for not being willing to help. My grandfather said he was tired of helping. I guess it had become a regular thing for years. This time he put his foot down and said no. My father couldn't buy the house without my grandfather's help.

He also might have been reluctant because my parents fought a lot. Mom started going out with friends once she started working and meeting new people. She was coming home later and later and going out more often. This one night I woke up from a chaotic noise coming from the kitchen. I ran out there to see what was going on. My mother had a large kitchen knife, like the biggest one in the drawer. She was going at my father with it. I without thinking jumped right in the middle of them. My father said to me, "Look what ya mother is doing ".

Although I was upset with my mother and afraid because she had a humongous knife in her hand. I was upset with my father as well because he let me stand in the middle of it. I guess he figured that she wasn't going to stab me, but she just might stab him. I get it, I guess there was no way out of that scenario clean. Shit I still have flash backs from it. There were a lot of situations like that.

My dad worked the third shift. He never took the new car. I think he was afraid of having an accident with it, because my mother loved that car so much. He took the bus to work every day instead. One time he was jumped by a bunch of punks while he was walking from the bus stop to work. He needed to walk through the city to get to his job. He carried a knife in his pocket from that point on. He wasn't safe at home or safe going to work.

My dad talked about the guys at work and the things there like the office pet, which was a vicious Snakehead fish. Every so often college kids would through laundry detergent into the fountain out in front of the building. He would turn the fountain off and laugh about the huge bubbles that floated around the city all night. He did seem to really like that job, or maybe it was just better than being at home. That's when you know life sucks!

Since my father was working third shift, my mother could pretty much do what she wanted. I was about twelve when my father picked me up from school and he seemed upset. He told me that he had to tell me something and that I couldn't repeat it. He was warning me that my mother had something to tell me after, and I needed to act surprised when she said it. He said that she was going to tell me that she's pregnant. The issue was that she wasn't pregnant by my father. I remained calm and was very strong for my dad. I didn't really react at all, I was frozen. He needed me, he was falling apart. This had to be the most painful thing he had ever gone through. I felt bad for him.

I saw my mother later that day and then she told me the news herself. I immediately burst into tears and cried my heart out. Nobody knew that she had been seeing someone. She said she was just going out with her friends. I knew instantly that it was going to be the destruction of my family.

When my father left for his midnight shift, Charlie came over. The father of the baby my mother was carrying. He would sleep over. I remember being in my bed and so scared because there was a strange guy in the house. Sometimes he brought a friend. My nerves always went right to my stomach. When I needed to use the bathroom, I would be so nervous that I'd just lay in bed all night suffering in pain. Never getting up to use the bathroom until the unfamiliar voices were gone.

A few times Charlie overslept and was still there in bed with my mother when my father got out of work in the morning. My dad saw the bicycle Charlie was riding in the driveway. That meant he was still there. My father just waited in the car outside of the house. He became a broken man. When I woke up and saw his car out there, I'd go sit with him while he was waiting for Charlie to leave. Charlie would eventually wake up and leave, riding off on his bicycle. I can close my eyes to this day and see it riding off. I personally don't know how my father didn't wake him up with a baseball bat to his legs, as the guys slept in his bed.

My dad moved out, and my parents got a divorce. I remember telling my mother that I wanted to stay with my father. I remember how hard it was to tell my mother that I didn't want to live with her, but she wouldn't allow it. Mom's new boyfriend Charlie moved in, and they immediately got married. I didn't want to stay, and I felt so bad for my father. I visited my father every day.

I was with him when he got the awful phone call. My dad's father, my only grandparent, had a stroke. This was devastating because he couldn't communicate anymore, and he lost the function of the entire right side of his body. It was sad. He was placed into a nursing home. The same nursing home that my mother worked in. My mother was good to him. No matter what unit she was working on, she would go to my grandfathers' room and always take care of him herself. She cared about him.

One day she was called into the office and was fired. She and her good friend Joline flashed their boobs to male patients a while back, prior to being pregnant. Not my grandfather either. They were getting a kick over how excited the old men got. It cost them their jobs though. My mother also was no longer there anymore to take care of my grandfather. The sad thing is I believe that my grandfather saw my mother with Charlie and didn't know my parents were separated. He probably saw it and suffered in silence because of the stroke he couldn't communicate.

There was a lot of back and forth. Some of it is a blur. Charlie and my mother didn't work out so well together. Charlie left, and they got divorced. My father came back and re-married my mother. Yeah, with my pregnant mother. He was with her for the whole pregnancy. At some point a sonagram showed that she was having twins. My father was willing to raise them both. He bought them cribs and everything else they needed. Charlie was gone for a while.

The day came that the twins were going to be born. It was a little early. They were premature. Dad and I were so excited to see the babies once they were born. My father accepted them, I did too. We went up the elevator and arrived at the hospital nursery. We stood there in front of the window anxiously waiting for the nurses to open the curtains. When they started to open, my father and I were in shock. My mother was sitting there with one of the babies, and Charlie was standing there with the other. This was after he had been gone, and my father was by her side the whole pregnancy. No warning at all. My father was devastated. He moved out again, this time I went with him.

I have always been an emotional fighter, because I was born into war. A battle within my own mind, fueled by my environment. With that being said, my dad and I were doing ok. My dad worked third shift, so he gave me his bedroom to use as an art studio, and a place to go build, create and try to enjoy my miserable life. He was making plans to fix the place up and make a small library area, he loved to read. He was planning to make it his own, with me by his side. I still liked to tinker with electronics. I had a table in one corner with my soldering iron and stuff like that. It was fun living peacefully with my dad. We did a lot, but we didn't have a car, so we walked... a lot.

I grew up with my parents listening to the HiFi stereo loud on the weekends. A little Pop music and a lot of Motown. My dad also loved Country music, like Willie Nelson and Waylon Jennings. This was the time when Rap music made its way from being underground to becoming popular. The only time I could listen to rap was on Sundays, from a local college station. With a blank cassette and tape recorder on hand, I'd record it all so I could listen all week and make mixtapes. Music became something that was, and still is important to me. Music has the power to shift my mood significantly. It is art.

I am Generation X; I was born into the birth of Rap. LL Cool J, and Run DMC were the first to catch my attention. I asked my dad for a big boom box, and I got one for my birthday. It was huge and it was loud. Critics thought that Rap was a fad that would fade away, but Rap/Hip hop became a Culture. Wearing Shell Top Adidas or Suede Pumas with fat laces, No matter what record store you walked into there would be a DJ spinning records. It was a good time to be a teenager during the birth of Hip hop. Then there was Graffiti. I painted the walls in my art room. Some graffiti made it to a few walls outside. I got caught tagging a wall near my school, and I got in a little trouble for that.

My father was struggling with the breakup from my mother and the scenario around that. He tried to hide it from me and take on living a single parent life. He tried so hard. I'll never forget when dad bought our first microwave oven. At first people thought anything could be cooked in it, and it could. But we soon learned that many things tase like crap. The market sold seasoning, which was also a coloring to spread over raw meat, like a chicken leg. It helped it look like it was cooked in an oven. That was exactly what my dad did. It was cooked, but it was gross. I ate it and told him it was good. I wouldn't dare hurt that poor broken man's feelings.

I must have showed signs of not taking it well because my father took me to therapist. I saw several over the years. One therapist told me straight out that I was damaged goods. That did not help. I will never forget that. I have seen quite a few different ones over many years. I learned to not really like therapists much. I felt they were just paid to listen. They really don't care, they're always looking at the clock that's often strategically located behind you, above your head. Maybe it was because they never seemed to be able to help my mother much, and that angered me.

I feel differently about it now. A therapist is a non-biased person who went to school to learn about the theory of people's minds. They also have experience with different people and all their different crap too. Talking to different people with different scenarios all the time. Getting a big snapshot of human behavior. So, they might be able to give some solid advice. I think it's great when you need someone to talk to and you don't have anyone else to listen. That's when you need therapy for sure. Family and friends don't always listen so well, at least in my case. Paying an experienced listener doesn't sound so bad.

I didn't truly know what pain was until I experienced death for the first time. I was drawing, and my father stormed into the house frantically. He had just found out that his dad died. My grandfather was a typical old timer. He still dressed like it was 1930. He wore dress pants, a button-down shirt, blazer, and a fedora on his head. His hardened face always looked a little miserable, but he was nice to me. He was the only grandparent that I knew. I loved him.

Before the stroke, and before he had the argument with my dad, I saw him once a month. My dad and I would go to his house to pick him up. I hated going into his house though, because he always had a lot of roaches. We brought him to his monthly doctor appointments, and we always went to Burger King right after. He stole the salt and pepper shakers off the table. He would literally take the salt and pepper shakers off the table and put them in his pocket. It's kind of funny thinking back on it now.

I could always count on him to give me a shiny quarter, twenty-five cents. I was a little kid, so I just took it and went to the candy store which was conveniently located right next door to the doctor's office. When Liam was still home, he was older and would get a dollar to spend.

The last time my father talked to his dad they argued and didn't speak for a while. Then he had a stroke, and it was too late to reconcile their differences. Then he was dead. That was his only parent, and he was once close to him. With all the heartache that had happened, my father was torn apart. He was trying to separate from my mother emotionally, and I can't say I blame him. He even tried dating, but it didn't work out, he just wasn't interested.

When my mother was living alone with my infant brother, and sister. I toggled between my parent's houses. My mother's mental health was declining rapidly. My father was slipping into a deep depression as well. I started to see signs that he was drinking a lot. I abandoned my own childhood and was totally engaged in my family's well-being.

There were a lot of situations. I often went to my mother's house after school to check on things. I walked into the house this one time and my mother was at the kitchen table slouched over. Twins were there too, both sitting side by side in their carriers facing her. No one in that room was aware but me. My mother was eating a raw potato like you would eat an apple and spooning sugar out of a bowl. She was eating it like it was a bowl of cereal. She was speaking as though she was a little girl. Finding miscellaneous foods was what she once did to survive as a kid.

She was in psychosis. It wasn't the first time, and it wouldn't be the last. I'm pretty sure I saved the babies' life that day. That one time sticks out so much because I thank God that I went there after school that day.

She was sitting in the chair the same way she did when she was little, Kris cross applesauce. Her voice became high pitched, different, almost like a split personality, but when she went into psychosis, she would appear to have a different personality at times. She talked to me as though she was a small child. It was frightening. I was petrified. Not for myself, but for the babies, and her for that matter.

I was trying to find a way to get her to the hospital. There was no rideshare back then. Family and friends became few and far apart as time went on. No one wants to deal with a crazy person, family or not. I ran down to the corner store and used the pay phone because our house phone was disconnected as usual.

I called my dad and for the first time he said, “No”. He wasn’t going to help her anymore. He was fed up. He left me to deal with her myself. I understood why, but I needed him to help me not her. I eventually got her to the hospital. She was still in a child state of mind and signed her name on the paperwork as though she was a preschooler, big letters and messy. it was her living life as a traumatized child again.

My mother was an emotional trainwreck. I was slowly deteriorating. Her mental health was out of control. Charlie wasn’t there, neither was my father anymore. My mother was in and out of the hospital so many times. There were so many suicide attempts, I lost track. Even though I was there every day to keep an eye on her, she was living alone with the babies for a short time. I also slept over when I was afraid for their safety, and that was often. Charlie’s parents took the twins while my mother was in the hospital getting better.

I had abandoned my own life fully. I tried so hard to take care of her. I always thought that she wasn’t sick like this when I was a little kid, but maybe I just didn’t realize it yet. Maybe when I was a little older, I started to see the differences. Although even as a kid I could see that she was different that the other moms I saw. It wasn’t like she didn’t try to get help either. She was always working on her mental health it seemed. Always going to therapist, psychiatrist, and neurologist. Nothing ever seemed to help.

It started to consume her, and she took on the labels she was given. Her title became a Manic Depressive, instead of a woman. She was more than likely predisposed to mental health issues, but with the shitty life she had to top it off, it's a miracle she made it as far as she did. It appeared that the more treatment she received and the more medication she was fed, the worse things became.

Her psychosis became challenging to live with. One night we went out to eat as a family, which didn't happen often. I was older, a young adult at least. She told the waitress in detail how her shoes were talking to her when she was cleaning out her closet the night before. After a while I avoided going in public with her as much as possible. Even though I lived it my whole life, I still didn't understand her fully yet, and it was embarrassing. I'm not bashing her; it is what it is. She is an important part of my story because **she created me**.

One night I woke up and I realized that my mother was not home, and I had no idea where she was. There were no cellphones yet. There wasn't even a house phone connected. The corner store was closed, so I couldn't go there to use the phone either. Even if I could, I don't know who I would have called. I was worried about her, and I just waited. She eventually walked in the door after a while. She was wearing a fur coat and a face full of makeup caked on way too heavy. I could usually tell the level of her mental health by how she was dressed, oddly enough. She was in bad shape.

I was relieved that she was home. She wasn't settling down

though. I was following her around and asking her questions that she wasn't answering clearly. I didn't know how she was getting around because she didn't have the car anymore since she sold the Mercury. She bought another one and almost killed herself hitting a telephone pole ironically like her mother. Either way she was on foot, and I figured she couldn't go far. I was relieved that she was home, but not for long unfortunately. She was packing a suitcase. I asked her where she was going. She was out of it, blacked out. Saying crazy outrageous things, but not where she was going.

I was franticly running back and forth begging her not to leave. It was in the middle of the night, early morning at that point. I noticed a strange car running out in front of the house. My mother was packing a bag to leave with this stranger. Packing like she was leaving for a while. I ran outside in the dead of winter in just my shorts. I remember because it was so cold. I begged this guy not to take my mother. I told him that she was very sick, and I was afraid for her. He looked at me and said, "She'll be fine".

I felt so defeated. I thought about what I could do to stop it, but there was nothing. I looked down at the ground and walked back into the house as I watched her leave. I didn't know if I'd ever see her again. I don't think I slept that night. She did return the next day. I never did find out where she went. Losing my mother was always a constant fear.

After all the countless hospitalizations my mother seemed to come back down to earth... a little bit. She divorced Charlie, and you guessed it. My father moved back in with her, and they remarried for the second time. She got the twins back and my father and her were raising them together. Charlie and his parents saw the kids on the weekends. My mother was more stable but never totally stable. She was eventually back in the hospital again. Charlie's parents kept an eye on the babies like they had in the past. The problem was that they didn't want to give them back this time, when she was feeling better. There was a vicious custody battle.

Mom's headaches were getting worse than ever. We made frequent trips to the ER for a shot to relieve the pain from her cluster migraine headaches. She was in so much pain that she would squirm out of her chair onto the floor. It was hard seeing her like that.

Chapter 6

Adolescence

We lived on Alverson Avenue for fifteen years. I basically grew up in this house. My favorite part was the attic, which was conveniently located off my bedroom. I spent most of my free time up there alone, drawing. I had my playboy magazine's hidden in the crawlspace above, and easy access to my parent's liquor where I had my first sip.

One time I had my buddy Josh sleeping over. We were sipping for the first time. It was late at night. We were hanging out the third-floor window where my art room was, drunk. Drinking and spitting the grossest stuff out the window as we were experimenting, discovering how terrible liquor tastes. The next morning, we went outside and realized that the neighbor on the first floor had their clothes hanging outside on the clothesline drying. The clothes were now covered with several different types of booze. We thought it was hilarious. I'm sure the neighbors didn't.

We did a lot of stuff together that one would consider rebellious. Without getting into his personal business, his life was challenging as well. We used to take apart fireworks and make bigger ones with the gunpowder inside, using a cigarette as a timer, among other stupid shit. We learned to shoplift. He stole mainly cassette tapes. I stole mainly computer parts and electronic components. I loved building things. I used to get schematic diagrams of electronic projects from the library. Then went and stole the components I needed to build them.

Neither of us were financially privileged. We both came from troubled homes, in different ways. He only had a mom, and not much money. I had my dad who worked and made okay money, but my mother's mental health always created a void preventing our family from ever progressing financially. Lots of memories in that house, good and bad.

As I got older, I didn't have many friends that I bothered with anymore, other than Josh. Through him I met his brother Jason who was a good kid. I became friends with them both. Somehow along the way my mother became friends with their mother as well. It was the first and only time that my mother hung out with a friend of mine's parent while I hung out with my friend. I was not little anymore either, so it was a little odd I guess. I would walk over to his house with my mother. She would stay downstairs with his mother, and I went upstairs with Josh and Jason. They had a little brother too.

One night my mother had said some inappropriate stuff to Josh's very religious, sweetheart of a mom. The moms weren't friends anymore after that. Josh and I started to not get along so well either. We were getting older and his mother very protective and wouldn't allow him to leave the house much and unfortunately, we drifted apart. We didn't speak again until we were young adults, early twenties.

I learned how to ride my bike a little older than most. For some reason I wasn't very interested. But once I got on that bike, I was gone. I'd take off with my friends and be towns away doing God knows what. I begged my parents for a very expensive Christmas gift that year, and to my surprise… I got it. It was a Freestyle bike, a GT Dyno. In the 1980s freestyling on bikes started to become popular but kept mainly underground at first. I got pretty good at it too. I spent all the money I could save upgrading the parts. It was beautiful, all purple and white with Mag Wheels.

I was great at surfing. I'd pedal as fast as I could down a long street to pick up speed. Then transition from sitting to standing on the frame, letting go of those handlebars. The bike was like a surfboard. It was a head turner. That bike became my freedom.

I also got stuck going to the market a lot as well. A good three-mile trip back and forth wasn't bad, except for the four bags a groceries that I had hanging off my handlebars. I didn't mind helping, but needing to carry so many bags with a car in the driveway could be annoying at times. I was respectful, I did what I was asked. I didn't even buy a snack with the change. I gave every penny of the change back.

With my wheels I became mobile and started making new friends. Until then the only friend I had over at the house was Josh. I rarely ever fought with anyone. I got along with almost everyone, except this one kid. He came by one day when I wasn't home. He was riding his bike up and down the driveway, antagonizing the little kid that lived on the first floor from us. He was being a jerk. My father got annoyed and told him to leave because I wasn't home. The kid replied to my father with, "Suck my dick". I went looking for him.

We met up and after a few swings back and forth I had him in a headlock and asked if he was ready to end it, I was satisfied, I defended my dad's honor. He said, "yes", and I let go. He turned around and sucker punched me in the face. I hit him once more time and ended it. His mother almost sued us because of the damage I did to his eye. I wasn't the type that went looking for a fight, but this kid deserved what he got.

His big brother came looking for me after that. He started swinging at me. I tripped and ended up on my back. He never got a good punch in though. My mother looked out the window and saw this big kid over me. She came up behind him and whacked him with a broom. I know she meant well, but it was embarrassing. The last thing a boy wants is his mom fighting his battles. That was the end of our friendship.

She seemed to always be around when I had friends over. It was strange and awkward at times. I was a teenager at that point. There was one awful night that's sticks out when I had friends sleeping over. We had a screened-in porch, and it was big enough for all of us to sleep out there all night. It was a hot summer night. We were having a good time and then there came my mother. She came out onto the porch and had a seat. She thought she wanted to hang out with us. We were teenagers, and I was filled with anxiety. Never sure what she would say or do next. I asked her to let us be and she became extremely upset. It was two o'clock in the morning and she sent everyone home. Their parents were furious to say the least. It was hard to live a normal life with my mother being so unpredictable.

It always seemed as though it couldn't get any worse, but then it would. Or maybe I was growing up and seeing things for what they really were. Either way I started to become more secluded. I started to abandon friends and was totally consumed with life at home. We would struggle financially, not because my father didn't make much money. He earned a decent living for that time. My mother would become Manic, and money would be mis-directed and spent wrong.

I have not so fond memories of people asking why the operator came on when they called me. I always said my phone lines were having issues. We spent plenty of cold winter nights huddled around the electric stove to keep warm because the heat had been turned off. My dad turned to the food bank and the church to help us get out of a financial mess at times.

My parents were friendly with the couple that owned the house we lived in. These two guys owned the house for a long time. They charged my parents less rent than they could have for the time. We lived there for thirteen years until they eventually put the house up for sale. They did want to sell it to my parents a little while back before the twins were born, but they weren't able to come up with the down payment. The new landlord purchased the house as a rental property investment. Our rent was raised significantly and apparently, we couldn't afford it. My parents went kicking and screaming though. We finally left by court order. We were evicted.

My mother made me draw on the walls and help her ruin the apartment. I was a smart kid; I just did what I was told. We then moved a few miles away to Atwells Avenue in Providence. It was on a main road and the neighborhood was pretty shitty. Not the shittiest, but shitty. We were going in reverse.

I was finally old enough to get a real job. I was almost seventeen. I started working for Baxter's liquors. It was a family-owned business. They had a few locations. I worked for this one in Providence. I got my friends jobs there too. There was a manager, and the assistant manager there who were characters to say the least. The manager was always high, selling drugs out of the place. Both the manager and assistant manager were stealing and setting a really bad example.

The assistant manager was an oddball. He was thirty-six years old and hung out with fifteen- and sixteen-year-olds. I hate to admit but we took advantage of him. Now that I'm older I can see he was just insecure and whatever else. I feel bad about it now because he was a nice guy. We were sixteen-years-old working at a liquor store. That shouldn't have been allowed in the first place. When it thundered out, he would leave us kids alone to take care of the liquor store by ourselves. While he was hiding in the basement.

There was an intercom system that he used to communicate with us from the basement. He'd say, "Let me know when the thunder is over". After he hadn't heard from anyone in a while. He checked in and we said, "Yeah, it's still pretty bad out". When in fact the sun had been shining for a while, birds tweeting, beautiful day. Keeping him down in the basement all day. We would drink and have a good time all day while we ran a liquor store at sixteen years old.

The store became a hang out spot after a while. We sold snacks and soda too. A lot of under aged kids frequented that store. This one girl named Rhonda kept coming in the store more than anyone else. She was almost sixteen. She used to come in and bother me. She started talking to me every shift, obviously flirting with me. She wasn't my type. I would talk to her, just to be friendly or whatever, but that was it. I was not interested in her romantically. People started telling me how much she liked me. This was a new experience for me. I had been cooped up in the house for a while before that. So, interest began to grow.

I had never been with a girl, but it was time. I figured that it was going to be easy since she already liked me. So, I didn't fear rejection. The last thing I needed was another challenge at the time. I was already emotionally exhausted from home life. I started talking to Rhonda more. She was cool to hang out with, and she was a girl. I started bunking school and hung out at her house. Her home was peaceful, comfortable and full of love. Their family bond became very attractive to me.

I missed a lot of my childhood fun dealing with family drama and at seventeen I was trying to be a normal kid. I had always worked hard, and it was hard to save money. My parents were often having a tough time. I was the kind of kid that helped out. This one Christmas my parents were dead broke. Not even a Christmas tree. I had a friend take me to a tree farm. I cashed my paycheck and bought my family the nicest tree I could find. I loved my family.

Things were so bad financially, huddled around the stove to keep warm. I considered holding up the convenience store down the street. The one that had the payphone I often ran to when my mother was in distress. I had compassion for my family, even with the cluster fuck of a life we had. I wanted to relieve their pain.

I was about to get my driver's license. My mother made me

wait until I was seventeen. I purchased my car stereo, subwoofers, and amps before I even looked for a car. I was so excited. I just wanted to enjoy being my age, which had been difficult to accomplish for so long. I went to work, and I went to school. I had already sacrificed so much of my childhood already. I wanted to spread my wings and fly. I needed to be able to escape.

I think about how dysfunctional life was then. I used to comb the house looking for sharp objects to hide, so my mother couldn't try to cut herself, and I did this for years. Ambulances, hospitals, and the musical husbands coming in and out. My father taking on kids that weren't his and pushing me aside. I was mad at my father, I felt like he abandoned me. I was getting older, but I was still a kid, and emotionally damaged. I still needed him, maybe more than ever. We started to not get along so well. He acted as though I wasn't important anymore and that hurt deeply. We were once very close. I felt as though I was there for him when the cards were down, and he didn't do the same for me.

My mother came to me one day, and I could tell she had something dramatic to tell me. I braced myself for the big news, or more likely, the bad news. My mother told me that my little brother and sister had been abused by their father. Not my father, their father, Charlie. I didn't know what to say. I knew my mother was a little off mentally, but she was very convincing. There were courts and lawyers. My mother was Spending all kinds of money, selling everything we had to pay attorney bills.

Over the years my father had four wishes. He always wanted to visit Nashville, get a motorcycle, and he always wanted a big oak roll-top desk. The only thing he ever got was the damn desk, and that was sold as well to pay attorney fees. There was conflicting evidence, as I was told. There was a spiral of events, none of which were good.

I was dragged into a courtroom full of people and put on the stand facing them all. I was asked questions, and I answered them to the best of my knowledge. I was not present for anything that was being discussed. I didn't know anything other than what I was told. Life was a mess. I was personally approaching becoming an adult and I wanted nothing to do with any of it.

Chapter 7

Life Changing Decisions at Age 17

I woke up one morning not knowing that I was about to make a life-changing decision that day. I was sitting on the floor drawing with my little brother, like we always did. I had so much built-up frustration over the years of turmoil that only seemed to get worse. They were so overwhelmed in the crappy life they had created together. I was no longer a priority.

My parents encouraged my art when I was younger. As time went on, they were focused on their failed relationship, babies and court battles. My future in art wasn't even a topic anymore. I became a damaged teenager who had just sacrificed his childhood to only be pushed aside afterwards and neglected. There was no time for any thoughts or discussions that pertained to me, unless it was to forbid me from doing normal teenager stuff.

They wouldn't let me drive my own car that I just bought and put music in. We moved away from the neighborhood I grew up in. That's where everyone I knew lived. I wanted to get away and be a seventeen-year-old. I was pushed away. There was no rideshare, without my car, I had no friends, and that meant being stuck in a house all day that was emotionally disturbing.

The drama at home had exhausted my patience. Arguing over the car, I threw the keys across the room, one of the keys got stuck in the door like a dagger. I sat there contemplating life and thought to myself, "I'm leaving". I knew my little brother would follow me. He was always by my side. I think back about it now. I feel really bad that I left him. I feel as though I abandoned him and my sister in that situation. I was just a kid myself though. Their lives probably would have been better if I had stayed there but unfortunately, I was at my breaking point.

My brother hadn't seen what I was doing because he was still drawing. I had given him a crayon and asked him to draw me something. Meanwhile I was packing. I went into my drawers and took one pair of Socks, underwear, T-shirt, and pants. I had one set of everything and the clothes on my back. I was working full time, so I knew I had a paycheck coming soon. I had a job making good money, working 60 hours a week.

When I say I ran away, I legit ran away from home. I snuck outside and ran. I dipped into driveways and hid behind bushes, looking back to see if they were coming to find me. I didn't want them to bring me back. I did this probably for about five miles. It was summertime at or around Rhonda's house when I wasn't working. I just needed a place to sleep. I contacted my father who had worked 3rd shift. Even though we had been arguing a little, we were always close in the past. He secretly took me to work with him at night. He had a spare room there with a kart for me to sleep on. It wasn't very comfortable, but it was better than going home. He never told my mother. He kept trying to get me to go home, but I told him that it wasn't happening. It wasn't him so much, it was my mother. He knew that. I went to work with my father for a few weeks and then I ended up talking to Rhonda's mother, and she let me stay there with them. I couldn't stay at my father's job forever.

I bought another car, because my parents wouldn't give me mine. I let it be because I felt bad, my car became the only car in the house. I found out later that they brought it to a mechanic to have the water pump fixed and abandoned it there.

I started working the third shift, so I only needed a place to sleep in the afternoon for a few hours. Rhonda's mother let me sleep there. My mother found out where I was. She called Rhonda's mother, asking her not to allow me to stay there. So, I would have to go home. My mother wasn't very nice about it though. After hearing a few of my war stories, Rhonda's mom let me stay, until I saved money and found an apartment of my own. I needed to buy a new car because my parents kept mine, which I worked on immediately.

My mother called child protective services to have them bring me back home. They came to the house to speak with me. I explained why I left. Basically, I couldn't deal with the insanity anymore, it was affecting my mental health significantly. As I became older, I was more aware that how I was living was not ok. Child protection said that because of my age, by the time it went to court, I would be eighteen. Legally allowed to make my own choices. They left and I stayed at Rhonda's. Nothing became of it. I was now starting my adult life early at the age of seventeen years old.

When I received my next paycheck, I went shopping and bought the essentials. I bought some clothes and I also bought paper, pencils, and markers so I could at least draw. I always loved art, but I wasn't educated about the job options that existed. When I was little my father told me to be a commercial artist, but I didn't know what that meant, and I didn't have the resources to explore opportunities. I loved art, it was who I was, and still am.

Regardless of any ups and downs, art was always present. I was petrified of being poor, always in survival mode. I became interested in robotics before Ai was a thing. Never giving up on art itself, robotic engineering was how I planned on paying the bills with. I saw art in that technology. If I knew the opportunities that were available in the world of art, I would have chosen that route ten times over, and it would have made me very happy.

I intended on going to college after high school. Perhaps I would have discovered opportunities in art or maybe I would have pursued robotics. I didn't realize that leaving home early meant sacrificing more than my own room. I was told that if I wanted to stay there at Rhonda's I would have to quit school and focus on work. I didn't want to do that, but I didn't want to go home with my parents even more.

There were two golden rules given to me... No being alone with Rhonda. Ronda was a virgin and her mother wanted to keep it that way, until marriage. The second rule was, don't drink the milk. It was for coffee. Rhonda's mom always had a huge commercial size coffee pot brewing, and everyone was welcome to swing by and grab a cup and maybe a little chat. There were always a lot of friends and family there.

We were young and her mom kept a close eye on us. I think she didn't want Rhonda pregnant and unmarried. So, we took advantage of every opportunity to be alone. That effort left me with scars for life. While we were babysitting her sleeping niece and nephew. We sat on a chair together in the living room, being teenagers watching TV. Her sister's cat charged at us from nowhere. One would think, "oh, just whack the cat off ya." That wasn't an option. I didn't see it coming, I was taken by surprise. This cat was circling our heads like you see in cartoons. Kind of funny now, but not so much then. My instincts were to cover Rhonda and shut my eyes as tight as possible.

I did finally whack the cat off us. I was surprised to not feel much pain, and I saw very little blood. I stood up and suddenly my face felt wet and was dripping blood. The dripping became fast and a lot. I looked in the mirror and at Rhonda. Our faces were sliced up. I could see the white fat cells in the open gashes on my face. No phone in the house, no cell phones yet either and we had two little kids with us. We held rags to our faces to hold back the bleeding and gathered the kids. There was blood everywhere. I remember clearly looking back at the floor and thinking that it looked like a murder had taken place.

We drove the kids to Rhonda's mother's house, and then we drove ourselves to the hospital. When we walked into the ER, the nurses thought we were in a car accident and our faces were cut by glass. Rhonda received eight stitches on her forehead. I received eighteen stitches around my right eye. It left me with scars. I have been self-conscious of it ever sense. I am grateful I didn't lose my vision that day though.

One thing led to another. A few months later, Rhonda's mother along with other family members were pushing for us to get married. "When you guys going to get married?", they pressed. I had nothing to lose, I was happier than I have been in a long time, if ever. I feared life at that moment. I was very attracted to her happy family. They all seemed to love each other so much and that was very appealing to me at that time.

Her family started organizing the wedding, making all the arrangements. We were just told how much things cost, and we paid for it. Rhonda's family helped too. I went out and bought affordable rings. After the damaged life I had been living, getting married became exciting at seventeen years old.

I was making decent money for my age but became a high school Dropout. I was smart, I missed most of tenth grade, yet I still graduated to the eleventh. At the time I really didn't know what I was doing. I was emotionally challenged, and I was getting married. I really didn't know what love or girls were even about yet. This was my first relationship ever. I don't think she really knew what she was doing herself. We were too young to make life decisions like that.

All I wanted was a stable place to call home. What I felt then I thought was love, maybe it was, maybe it wasn't. I don't know. I was too traumatized by the time I left my parents' house. I look back and I can now see how vulnerable I was. The saddest part is that my parents weren't there to see me get married. There was nothing they could do to stop it though. I was not going back home, it wasn't happening. I understand why they were so concerned; but they were also blind to see what was chasing me out of the house in the first place.

A day after my eighteenth birthday Rhonda's mom took us to city hall, so we could get our marriage license. Rhonda wasn't eighteen yet, so her mother signed the paperwork and gave her permission to get married, also emancipating her at the same time. I never really understood why she would want to condone her sixteen-year-old getting married. As a parent myself now, the normal thing a parent would do is try to stop it, and not encourage it. I guess she had her reasons, she must have.

Now that I look back at it, Rhonda was her youngest kid, and to be honest she wasn't doing so well either before we met. At fifteen-sixteen years old she was doing more than smoking weed. I encouraged her to be better. Her mother did not know this of course I thought at the time, but she probably was aware. Her mom must have seen that her daughter had a chance at a decent life with me. Or maybe I am wrong.

A week after my 18th birthday we got married. We didn't have anything in common, other than being each other's first. She had already done little shit that showed she wasn't very trustworthy. We didn't really enjoy each other's company as much as a newly married couple should. I was more mature, and she acted her age. I think she felt persuaded too. I was a good catch for her, coming from where she was at. For me, it was an escape route. In a way we needed each other at that time in our lives. I believe everything happens for a reason.

The family bond they all had was attractive. I was so screwed up; I didn't even think I knew other options existed. She liked me; it was easy. I didn't even know what love was. I certainly never experienced seeing it at home. My father was more of a father figure to my mother.

Looks are not everything for sure. What we see on the outer surface is temporary and it changes as the years move on. The only control we have is taking care of ourselves the best we can and learning from our experiences. Everything on the inside, that's for life. I don't think that we weren't really attracted to each other on the inside, the way two people getting married should be.

We were too young to understand something as serious as marriage. We had our first apartment. I had it by myself for a few months before we got married. Once we were married Rhonda moved in too. I was the only one working and making decent money at that time, especially for a kid. I was setting goals and working hard. Life was a lot less expensive in 1989. It was a lot easier to afford life then.

I planned to work hard, save money, and make a go at life. I was very mature for my age. I think she was still very immature yet. It wasn't her fault though, after all we were only teenagers. I had seen a lot growing up, so that is what matured me quicker. I missed out on most of my childhood., and she was kind of still living hers.

Rhonda's mother started questioning me about kids, and why we weren't planning any yet. I told her that I was only eighteen, and I wanted to be better established first. Her reply was, "What are you shooting blanks, you'll figure it out". She was serious but funny about it. I didn't know that then though. I took it serious, she was aggressive about it.

I was already an emotional mess, and this was not helping at all. I was very vulnerable at that time, and I don't think she understood the severity of it. Why and how would she. She was a comedian; I was lacking a sense of humor then. I was a very serious person. I was just a fucked-up kid.

BAM! My first child was on its way. Once it happened, I was happy. I was going to make the family that I dreamed of. I was petrified because there was a war starting in Iraq, and this was the first war in my adult life. I was worried the draft would return, and I wanted to be home when the baby was born.

Rhonda's mom was a good person, I learned to love her like a stepmother to be honest. She could also be tough; she had a difficult life herself. She was adopted, and then both of her adopted parents died in a car crash together. She had a hardness to her but would do anything for anyone. I respected her. We would sit at the kitchen table, talking late at night over a cup of coffee. just her and I. She confided in me with topics that she didn't share with anyone else. She trusted me. She also saved me from an abusive environment too, so I trusted her as well. She treated me like a son.

I love my son very much. I clearly remember the day he was born. I was in the delivery room of course. The baby was a boy, and I was the first person to hold him. My first thought was that he looked like me. I counted all his fingers and toes just like my mom did with me when I was born. It was very emotional. I was super excited that I had a son. I instantly had a whole new outlook on life. Someone else was more important than myself now, and that was okay with me. Unconditional love... I'll take it! I was a damn good father, especially for a teen dad. Boy did we struggle. I remember eating dry coco out of a can of hot chocolate powder. Rhonda's family were generous and did help with things they were able to.

The third shift job I had was because my dad knew a guy and he helped me get it. I was working for a company, retro fitting commercial lighting to be more energy efficient. I was limited to what I could do because a lot of work was on twenty-foot ladders at times, and I couldn't climb ladders that high I found out soon after. Work went from sixty hours a week to twenty, so it didn't last much longer. I did make a few friends there and help my brother-in-law Devin out who was a good guy and had a tough life. He really needed the job and had a family. He embraced that opportunity and did well. That made me feel good, but I had to move on.

It was Christmas time. I ended up working part time in two different retail stores in the same mall, a Toy store, and a big department store. My shift at the department store ended at three o'clock, the same time my shift at the toy store began. I was fortunate that they allowed me to be a few minutes late. That allowed me enough time to literally run there from the morning job at the department store.

Both jobs required Khakis, a button-down shirt, shoes and a necktie. I had one of each, right down to the one red necktie. The same one I wore to my wedding. I did what I had to do. Things were so tight that I could only go grocery shopping when I had over-time from working Sundays, which was every other week. I was the primary provider. I worked hard as a seasonal employee at both stores. To my surprise, both jobs wanted to keep me after Christmas ended. I decided to stay at the toy store. With this opportunity for my new family, I worked even harder and tried to learn as much as possible. Within that year I became the assistant manager at nineteen. I wasn't earning much, but I always worked hard. We barely got by. I was nineteen years old supporting a family of three.

Chapter 8

Encountering Opportunities

I was working in retail at the toy store. It wasn't what I had planned for a career, but I had mouths to feed. After a while I was transferred to a different mall, which is common in retail. This transfer was going to be a game changer for my future, not in retail, but with art. Until then I did a lot of drawing, but that was the extent of it. I was focused on providing and getting by week to week at nineteen years old.

I was at work, standing at the register area of the store one day. I was watching a new retailer move into what was until then an empty kiosk right outside the toy store. Naturally I was curious to see what was moving in. Then I saw that he was doing the coolest thing I'd seen in a while. It was new to me. He was an airbrush artist. I was amazed at the concept. I visualized new opportunities and things that could be done with this new-to-me medium. For the first time I saw an opportunity to make money with art, like this guy was doing. I was home with friends one night and I started talking about this airbrush guy I saw at work. I wanted to try it too, but I could not afford the equipment that looked expensive. My friend said his brother had an old airbrush that he didn't use.

I didn't have extra money, but I had a small collection of knives that he was interested in. I traded the knives for the airbrush. I cheaply rigged together a medal air tank that I filled up with an electric tire air pump, which was a gift from Rhonda's aunt. The air tank would empty fast, but it worked. I taught myself how to airbrush.

I started airbrushing t-shirts first because that was the only thing I saw being done. I immediately started making money. There was no You-Tube yet, I taught myself with practice and books from the library. Quickly I had people paying me to make them custom shirts and pants. My district manager at the toy store found out I was an artist and commissioned me to make a bunch of shirts for a manager meeting he was having. I started airbrushing a lot and was getting a bunch of work to do. I was making much needed money at it.

I did not realize then, all the paths the introduction to airbrushing would take me with art. I was transferred to a new store and the manager didn't like me so much. I eventually lost my job at the toy store. Airbrushing became my only revenue. God works in mysterious ways. I was still able to provide.,

Rhonda started to display some red flags. I mean she had started adult life too young; I get it. She wasn't ready. I see that now. We were just kids. It was all too much for us, but she went too far. She started hanging out with the kid across the street and his cousin. I was inside with my son. Sticking my head out the front door, yelling for her to come in. She ignored me.

We were young, like twentyish, but still a family. She was a married mom hanging out with a group of boys at two o'clock in the morning. Laughing at me as I tried to take care of a two-year- old and convince his mother to come home.

This was my life, and it seemed as though Rhonda was cheating on me. My grandfather's wife was caught with another man, my father had two marriages where he delt with woman leaving him. Now it was happening to me. My mother always told me to never trust a woman. In retrospect that was not good advice, but at that point... she wasn't wrong so far. I had just left home a few years prior. This situation was tweaking me out.

I tried hard and never gave up too easily. I was being tested. I was getting attention from other girls. I was very young, and Rhonda made it extremely difficult to ignore the fact that I had options too. I was angry with Rhonda and hurt, as I left her. Looking back at it now, I understand better, we were just young, but neither of us handled our young minded confusions well. We both made mistakes. I was gone for a few days, but I saw my son daily. Not being with him was tearing me up. I couldn't stay away.

Rhonda saw her mistakes and didn't want to break up. What I really wanted was my family. I wanted to tuck my son in at night and be there when he woke up in the morning. Rhonda said that she wanted to make it work, and things were ok for a while. Or what our version of okay was then. A year later my daughter Tammy was born. She was beautiful. I adored my little girl. I was happy to have a son and a daughter too. I was close to my kids and a good dad, especially for being a kid myself, who was raised in a dysfunctional environment. Tammy used to get so excited when she saw this one commercial. It was for a new doll that kids could put tattoos on. She would dance and giggle, she loved that commercial.

She was so cute in her little pink head band. She ended up being nicknamed after the doll. The name stuck with her for life. I wasn't fond of the name Tammy. I was too quiet then to make a big deal over it, so I accepted it. One of my fondest memories with Tammy was getting home from work every day and pulling into the driveway. She ran window to window yelling, "Da-e Da-e". Trying to say daddy.

I Airbrushed at festivals in the summer and flea markets in the winter. I made a living from it for a few years, I wasn't rich, but I supported my family. The largest commission I've ever received was from ESPN when I painted a twenty-two thousand square foot skating platform. It was covered with ramps and half pipes. Big names in those sports were there. I was painting right up until airtime.

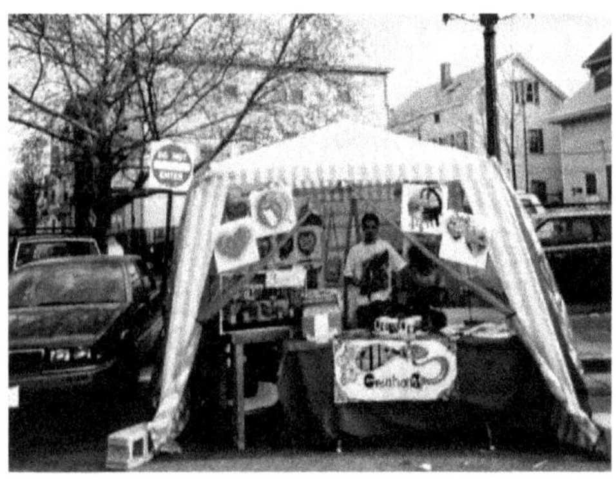

Providence, festival airbrushing (1996)

The final moments before it aired live on TV I was still painting. There were a few tire tracks made from paint being wet right up until airtime. It was the ESPN X-Games, and my work was on TV all week. I was and still am proud of that accomplishment. I completed this job with my good buddy Jimmy. Rhonda and my brother-in -law helped as well. I had a routine going after a while, festivals during the summer. I would pick up work to do during the week as well. During the winter I did the same thing but at the flea market. It may sound shitty, but it was paid the bills and fed us.

Soon after pagers, otherwise known as beepers, became popular and mainstream in the early 90s. They were huge before cellphones became a regular thing. I discovered that I could airbrush the pagers, and people loved that. I did pretty good for a while, because it was unique. I was making decent money, enough to provide. I was a full-time dad, and I had a business. I was a professional artist, earning money, paying the bills and feeding the family with my God given talents. I thought it could only get better from there.

Chapter 9

Fork In the Road, My20s

Airbrushing at a flea market is when I met Jimmy. He came up to me and started to admire my airbrush work. He was very friendly. He began to tell me that he knew how to get all the cable channels for twenty bucks. It was random. At the time it was a great deal. He had a device that sent a signal into the cable box. I was like, "Yeah, ok, Let's do it".

He drove over to my house the next day. He pulled out a little black box and put it next to my cable box and pressed a button. BAM! I had all the channels. He told me he'd be back because once a month the box would need to be reset.
For whatever reason we vibed well and he stayed for a while. He just hung out with me, and we talked and talked. Then he came over again the next day. Within no time we were hanging out every day. We just instantly got along well. He was a few years younger than me, he was a senior in high school, but very mature. He had an old soul.
I was with Rhonda when I met Jimmy. He started to come over early in the morning after a while. I'd hear a knock on the sliding glass doors, and it was Jimmy. I let him inside and

he slept on my couch until I woke up for the day. It was whatever. It went on for a little while.

I started to realize that this kid was here way too much. He was in his senior year of high school, and he obviously was not attending school. I told him I wasn't going to let him in the house if he came over instead of going to school again. "So, go to school", I said to him. He listened to me. He respected me, I guess. Not only did he go back to school, but he made the honor role for the first time. He graduated from high school. He told me that he graduated because of me. He was very smart. At first, I was like Jimmy's big brother. As time went by, we became best friends. We were close, like TV show best friends.

Shortly after, Rhonda and I bought a house. It was in her mom's name tentatively because I didn't have sufficient proof of income. I recently opened a new business with Jimmy. I was a hustler, trying to live comfortably and be a good provider. We moved into this new house in the pouring rain, I'll never forget. That summer I tore up the yard and installed a pool, rolled out fresh green grass, and built a play area with a swing set. I gave my two kids the best backyard I could create for them.

When Jimmy graduated, we opened the store together. It was prime time for pagers, everyone had one, and cellphones were starting to make their way too. The profit was great. I continued to Airbrush beeper cases for other stores in Rhode Island and Massachusetts. As well as owning my own brick and mortar retail store. Art was always part of my life in one way or another, no matter what I was doing at the time. Jimmy and I were partners. He introduced buying and selling gold to the business. We basically had two businesses within one four wall establishment.

This kid Bobby from the neighborhood was in and out every day. His mother was a drug addict and prostitute unfortunately to get by. He was a smart kid, brilliant. The first time we saw him he walked into the store wearing nothing but his boxer shorts asking if we were hiring. He was persistent and we eventually gave him a job. He was a good kid that needed guidance.

I was finally doing pretty good. With a new house, and a new car after I taught Rhonda how to drive and somehow, she took my Grand Am for a drive and it caught on fire in a parking lot. I had just finished paying that car off. I replaced it with a new car for Rhonda and picked up a crappy shitbox to get back and forth to work in for myself. I was busting my ass to have a profitable business. Hard work was finally starting to pay off. I had struggled ever since I left home at seventeen.

Then one day I went to open the store and someone from the neighborhood said, "Rhonda is fucking around with Jack". I laughed and said, "Get the fuck outta here, there's no way". See, Jack was not a guy, he was a sixteen-year-old kid. I was doing pretty good for a young guy, especially with the difficult start I had. Plus, we had two kids together, a home etc. We were a married couple.

I was busting my ass to make a better life for my family. Also dealing with major debilitating anxiety, that I didn't quite understand yet at that time. The day came and I found out it was true. It was Jack's brother Jason, for some reason he had finally confirmed it to me. I think they were beefing maybe. They were young kids. Jason called me one day to tell me where Rhonda and Jack were, so I could catch them in the act. I guess I needed to see it, to truly believe it. Especially when we were doing so well. Obviously, not too well. I just didn't see it. I was too busy trying to make life better for us.

I raced up to where they were supposed to be going. I took a few people, because I knew they were with a few people too, who would certainly get involved. I got there and they were gone. I missed them. I drove back down to the neighborhood still looking for them. At this point it was just me and Jimmy. I was so upset! Finally, at 2 am I saw the little Hyundai. The car that I bought for Rhonda.

I raced up to him with fire and hatred in my heart. They took off at full speed, in the car that I was paying for. I flew past them, and Jack was driving the car. It was like a scene from an action movie. I raced past them and blocked the car off. I blocked the road so that he couldn't go anywhere. Their car doors swung open, Jack and his friends jumped out. They took off! Rhonda was left in the back seat speechless. I could not find them, as they were hiding in yards. I wanted to kill this kid. I'm glad I didn't find him, because I would have gotten in trouble that night if I did.

He used to hang around my store and act like he was cool with me. In fact, when he's with my wife on the side. He screwed himself. He was a kid that didn't know what he was doing. I see that now. It was her bad, really. Of course, when this first happened, I hated him. I was devastated! I gave her a chance to come back, and she did. The very same night I couldn't find her anywhere, until I did. She was hiding in the basement talking on the phone with Jack. I bugged out and threw all her clothes on the front porch. Her mother was so disappointed in her too. I reached my boiling point.
Rhonda was couch hopping again and staying at hotels. First

with my money. She was carrying around bags with clothes and essentials. I had the kids; her mom was helping me so I could work. I wanted legal custody because she was clearly not capable of being a mother at that time. Her mom was backing me up with full support. I asked Rhonda to sign full custody over to me. She did it. I got temporary full custody. Nothing goes without cost though... I met her at the attorney's office, and she signed. She was going to sign permanent custody over to me later. She was negotiating with me, she wanted money.

She was always asking for money. She came to my store this one time asking me for money. She and Jack probably needed to get a room. They were roaming the streets like kids but needed a place to sleep at night. I refused and she flipped my store upside down. I had to go to court and ask for a no contact order against her. It was embarrassing. I was the only man in the room courtroom. I was trying to protect my business, that fed the kids.

I told Jimmy one night to bring over some weed. I said, "I want to smoke." He said, "You sure?" I said "ABSO-FUCKING-LUTLY"! It was my first-time smoking. Weed was still taboo at the time. Against the law even. I can remember it like it was yesterday. I heard a knock on the door. When I opened the door, there was Jimmy with a big fat blunt in his ear. He said, "You ready?" I went outside, and we went for a walk-up the Street.

I'm puffing this blunt he brought over, passing it back and forth. I told him that I didn't feel any different. He replied with, "You will, just keep smoking ". Then it finally hit me. I had the time of my life. If I made a list of most memorable moments in my life... that moment would be on that list. We just talked and joked. We laughed our asses off and made cinnamon toast bread. First time I ever had the munchies. It was the best toast I had ever eaten in my life.

So, we're sitting outside chilling on the front porch. This guy Toby pulls up. He went by Lil' T. He was not little at all. He drove a Harley and was affiliated with a motorcycle club; I'll leave it at that. Nicest guy ever though. Were blazed up at that point. Me and Jimmy watched him pull up and he just looked at us. Jimmy and I looked at each other and we just started laughing our asses off. He looked at us and said, "What's so funny". Then he realized what was going on. He said," You smoked for the first time". He was so excited to have been part of it. It was a memorable night. We all laughed hard. Just having a good time. From that night on I never stopped smoking. It helped anxiety, sleep, appetite and depression.

Rhonda had a change of heart. Her mom came to me and said that Rhonda wanted a chance to be a mom again. She was supporting her daughter now of course. This was in the 90s. It was nearly impossible to get custody unless the mother was beating her kids senselessly. A lot had happened, and all I was concerned about was the kids. I gave Ronda two hundred dollars for a hotel room. I gave her the car, and the family photo albums. I wanted her to really think about what she wanted that night. She took the money and the car. She picked up Jack and spent the money on a hotel for them both instead.

Those photo albums never made it out of the trunk. There was no saving it, it had all gone way too far. I immediately found a lawyer so I could start planning and paying child support voluntarily. I wanted to be sure I was able to see my kids without issues. At the time I was still paying for a lot of other things as well. I'm pretty sure that the kids were not aware I even contributed at all.

I filed for a divorce. Rhonda tried to stop me. Sent me flowers and a heartfelt card. It went too far. Jack's age is what got to me, he was a child. I thought how bad was i... that a child was better than me, her husband. We were getting a divorce, and she was mad. I guess she wanted to keep her quality of life with me and still have fun on the side. I ruined that for her. I felt as though I sincerely tried. I gave her more chances than most guys would have. More chances than she deserved, really. She moved back in with the kids, as I moved out. She was young, but so was I.

Jimmy and I spent a lot more time at the store, and we even got an apartment together. We were living right upstairs from my parents. I think deep down inside I was vulnerable and damaged from everything that had just happened. Being closer to my parents helped ease the pain. I found ways to occupy my free time with parties, and girls. I was in my early twenties. I spent time on art, which has always been part of what I do. I did all I could to get through each day without my kids, Monday through Friday. I was doing my best to make life doable. I started self-medicating.

I escaped the anxieties of my parents' home a few years back and was trying to have a loving family of my own, and I gave it my best. It just didn't work out, and there were no signs at all that it could ever get better. I didn't fight to keep the marriage because I knew that it was beyond that. We would be dealing with these types of situations forever, I gave up. Besides having my kids on the weekends and paying child support. I took care of whatever else they needed, shoes, jackets, etc. Whenever I could afford it. I knew Rhonda didn't have a lot, and the kids weren't going to see much of that child support money. I paid it faithfully every week though. I took them places... Amusement parks, movie theater, water parks, beaches, playground, camping... we did a lot.

Rhonda made things hard. If I was sick, she didn't believe me. She would tell the kids that I didn't want to see them. Maybe that's what she really thought. Being a dad living in a separate home is emotionally challenging. Unless you have a good relationship with the mom, you will often be made to look like a bad guy.

I agree whatever child support most men pay isn't enough, even what I paid. On the other hand, imagine putting hundreds of dollars a month into a house that you don't live in and still try to keep a roof over your own head and food in your stomach too. You come out more broker than broke, still looked at as not doing enough! Often coming out looking like a villain even when your intentions are not bad at all. It just is the way it is. A man's value is unfortunately measured by their ability to provide and capability to sacrifice.

I couldn't understand why I was the bad guy. She was the married woman messing around with a teenage boy. I never wanted to lose my kids. In fact, I wanted to keep and raise them myself. I was always present, I never disappeared. I paid and bought what I could. I really tried my best. Yet I was always looked down on, as I could have done better. A lot was expected of me at a very young age. I never had a childhood, I didn't get to enjoy the experience of being a teenager, and then I wasn't able to enjoy being a daddy to my kids either, living in a different house. None of these situations were self-inflicted. I just kept getting screwed!

When I filed for a divorce, she sent me flowers and thought that I would take her back again. I had already tried several times. I think she thought I was bluffing, and she could string me along. She thought she could have fun and come back to a safe place or maintain both lives maybe. She was mad that her plans were ruined. Shortly after I was dating pretty girls and living my life. Still being the best father possible. Trying to make the best of things. On the surface it looked like I was ok moving on. In all actuality I was damaged beyond repair.

I cried my eyes out every Sunday after bringing the kids home. I had a broken heart. Not because Rhonda was gone so much. I was angry with her, and I lost what feelings I had left. My broken heart was because for the first time I was not able to tuck my kids into bed at night. I wasn't there when they woke up in the morning and no longer eating dinner with them. A different person was doing that now, a kid who was sixteen. I had no idea how he was treating them. I was defeated on so many levels.

They were two and five years old. I missed out on their milestones, victories and defeats. I was already a broken man. I was falling apart rapidly. I couldn't even give Jack too much shit because he was a sixteen-year-old kid. I had to swallow my pride. I now had to get through the week without my kids. Jimmy became a significant part of my life; I am not sure how I would have gotten through it without him. Jimmy saved me and was corrupting me at the same time. Sometimes shit happens for a reason.

We were together each day during the week. He knew I was having a tough time and was a true friend. Jimmy and I went to a strip club from time to time. Not to drool over naked girls, but just to have a few drinks and be around girls. One night after the club closed, we left with two dancers and went to a 24-hour breakfast place. Right behind me as I was in line with Jimmy and two dancers... Rhonda, with a couple of her friends. It was a satisfying moment. Even though I was a mess inside, she saw that I was pulling good looking girls and I looked like I was having a good time. We went out, we had fun. Jimmy was known to have a little too much fun at times. We drank a little, we smoked, and then Jimmy introduced cocaine into the mix.

One day Bobby was having issues with a guy bothering his girlfriend. He asked Jimmy for a ride to meet up with this person. I believe that he had every intention of fighting. Marvin was an old friend of mine and was hanging out with us as he often did. We all hopped in Jimmy's car, and I paused. I knew that Jimmy had cocaine on him. Nobody used any of it, but driving with it was a bad idea. I said, "Stop, wait, put that inside before we leave ". He thought that I worried too much, but he listened to me.

Jimmy was driving and passing by a playground. What seemed like out of nowhere, a kid ran out from in between two parked cars. Jimmy hit the brakes and skid right into a four-year-old child. I can remember the sound I heard when the kid's head contacted the car bumper. It was a hard thump and I'll never forget that sound. As fast as it happened, I saw it all happen in slow motion. I saw the kid fly up in the air and land on the ground. I screamed and ran out of the car. I put my coat over the little boy. He wasn't moving and we thought he was dead.

We were young and driving a Mustang GT 5.0. Within seconds there was a crowd of people about to tear us apart. They understandably were assuming that we had done something wrong. Thankfully, the police arrived quickly. We stayed at the police station all night being interrogated. I could hear Jimmy throwing up in the next room. Cops were telling us that the little boy might die because his brain was swollen. It was frightening.

My son was four-year-old too, so it hit home big time. Thankfully the little boy made a turn for the better and lived. I don't know if he had any injuries that would affect him long term. I just know he lived. His mother tried to sue Jimmy, but she lost because she admitted that she wasn't paying attention to her child. Jimmy was driving and wasn't speeding. It was just an unfortunate accident.

It was a traumatic experience for everyone involved, to say the least. It was the last time I saw Marvin for a long time. He was one of the nicest kids I ever knew. A genuinely good guy, I missed him. That Christmas Jimmy bought the biggest swing set he could find, and had it anonymously delivered to the kid's house. The family must have known it was from him. Regardless of whose fault, he felt terrible. We all did. He was never the same after that to be honest. Nothing really was. I get a sick feeling when I drive by that park to this day. I feel like that was a turning point for us all.

"Trust in the Lord with all your heart, and do not lean on your own understanding. In all your ways acknowledge him, and he will make straight your paths."
Proverbs 3:5-6

Chapter 10

Epiphany

I only had a few friends besides Jimmy, who himself knew a lot of people. He introduced me to new people over time. I made a lot of new acquaintances. One of those people was Jess. I talked to a few girls after Rhonda, nothing serious. Jess liked me a lot and I liked her. She was a hell of a lot nicer to me than Rhonda was, and she was an attractive girl. She was also very understanding with what I was going through emotionally with everything that had happened. She became my second long-term relationship.

I started spending more time with Jess. Jimmy wasn't crazy about it. He wanted us to be chilling and having fun, where I was trying to figure out life. She came from a good, solid family, sort of privileged. She was a different kind of girl than I was used to. It was nice. She saw how low my self- esteem was and helped me get through the difficult times. She was supportive, and she kept me away from risky situations. Deep down I was a quiet guy who really enjoyed being a dad. I was a peaceful person but felt defeated by life. I was trying to survive and occupy my time between weekends when I didn't have my kids. Jimmy started to do things that were more dangerous that I didn't want to do. He brought dangerous people into our business and our lives. Plotting crimes that would have gotten us decades in prison if caught. Some things that I wouldn't have been able to live with myself afterwards.

He was disappointed that I wasn't interested. He asked me if I was afraid to go to jail. I said, "absolutely". Then he said, "I don't give a fuck". There were a few close calls. Thats when I took a step back and separated myself. It was tough because Jimmy and I were extremely close, closer than blood. Things were getting dangerous with the lifestyle he started taking on. I saw myself doing things that I would never have done before. It hadn't gone too far yet, but I needed to nip it in the bud before it was too late.

We had business together, we lived together, and we hung out together. I Just woke up one morning with the thought in my head that enough was enough. It was like enlightenment, a moment of clarity...an epiphany! I don't know if I had a dream that prompted this, but I woke up with a whole new outlook on life. I didn't have my kids Monday through Friday, but I was still their dad. I needed to keep my life together, so I was always able to be there every Saturday through Sunday. I was gonna have to make some serious changes. I didn't even open the business that day. I put a sign in the window and just started to break things down. Jimmy was extremely upset about it.

At first, we were two single guys having a good time but then it started getting a little carried away. I had a lot of good times with Jimmy. If you hung out with him, it was a guaranteed good time. Too much fun is not good though. If he went down a different path and tried to put more effort into a positive life. He could have gone so far. He could have been a standup comic. He would just walk into the room and make you laugh by looking at you. He had that face. I used to encourage him all the time, but he said that he couldn't do it on command. It was extremely hard because I loved him like a brother. I walked away and missed him dearly. It was a life-or-death situation.

Missing someone is not reason enough to keep them in your life, especially a friend. I hadn't seen him for several years. He moved out of state which one would think was an attempt to turn his life around too. He moved to North Carolina, and shortly after he ironically was sentenced to two years in jail. He made a new best friend down there who was also a quiet clean-cut mature guy, and this guy Harry had his life together, unlike myself. Within a year I found out that Harry was found dead on the bathroom floor with a needle in his arm. I realized then that I saved my own life!

I was going through a lot emotionally, and I was vulnerable as fuck at times, but I saw the signs. If I didn't make that hard decision and separate myself as I did, I might be dead myself right now too or in prison. Life is all about choices. One bad choice and your life is over. I am lucky to be alive!

After I closed my business and removed all the negative aspects of my life, as much as possible. I was still dealing with Rhonda who gave me a hard time. One day she asked me to sign my rights to my kids over to her boyfriend. There was no way I would or could ever give up my children like that. No matter how awful Rhonda made life for me. I was told many years later that she told my kids that I requested to sign them over. The 100% absolute opposite. I got a raw deal and

I never truly understand why. Things were challenging, it seemed like things were always that way.

Art remained a big part of my life. I originally started airbrushing art on paper and then canvas. I liked it. Then I bought some paint brushes and tubes of acrylic paint. I started mixing airbrush work with regular brush work. I was practicing and learning. I was reaching for my artistic direction. One of the hardest things as an artist is trying to find your style, but You can't find it; it needs to find you!

My son was a little older when his mother and I split up, and we were close because of that. He remembered when I still lived with him. I'm sure he had questions over the years that he never asked. A really shitty situation. Tammy was so young all she knew was what she heard from others like her mom. She was once close to me and then became always so quiet. It was upsetting. I did the best I could with the whole situation. All one can do is put in the effort and thrive for a better today and tomorrow.

I was broken than broke, I sold off everything I could from my closed business. I had no source of income; Jess had a part-time job. Things were getting tough. Jess and I moved in together and had bills to pay. I didn't know what I was going to do. I had a box of blank white pager cases left over from the store. It had been months since I airbrushed any. I was close to rock bottom.

I took the blank white cases I had and created twelve new designs and made a sample of each. I took a picture of them and made a flyer that I sent to every pager store within an hour's drive. I waited a day for the mail to be delivered, and the phone rang. More calls came in every day. I was lucky, becoming the sole designer, creator, and distributor of all the airbrushed pager cases in the surrounding area. It worked!

I started making them for a distributor in New York who sold them all over the country. I progressed and added a line of accessories to my catalog. I was self- employed and supporting myself once again and embracing art at the same time.

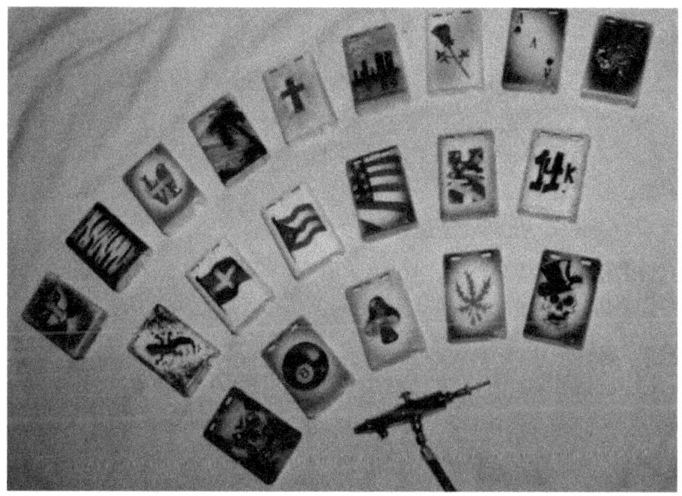

Airbrushed Beeper cases (1996)

It was just Jess and me. I had abandoned every friend I had. Because once I stepped back and saw the path I just dodged, I was petrified and thankful. I was grateful that I removed myself from the cycle I was slipping into. I would sure be sorry about after if I didn't. One person that was impossible to avoid was Bobby. He was the kid that we hired at the store. His family life was so bad, and he had nobody that cared. He found me quickly and lingered. I felt bad, and for what it was worth, he was a good friend thus far. He looked up to me and respected me. I tried to teach him a better way to live.

Many have a teacher that stood out in their life for whatever reason. For me that was Sister Smith, my teacher during a challenging time in my life when my mother was in and out of the hospital. She consoled me and even went to visit my mom. She was my guardian angel. We wrote back and forth for years and stayed in touch. After my divorce with Rhonda, Sister Smith happened to be taking a trip back to the United States. She was visiting a convent in Newport. She was living in Canada where she was originally from. We made plans to meet up.

When I arrived at the convent, it was surreal. It had been a long time since I saw Sister Smith. We sat out on the back deck and talked, surrounded by beautiful scenery overlooking nature. She was so angelic. If I found out she was never a real person, and just an angel watching over me, I'd believe it. She introduced me to a frail old lady who was also a nun. She was referred to as Mother. She was dying, yet in so much at peace. It was a deep, humbling moment that I am privileged to have experienced.

Back home, Jess and I were close for the first six months or so. Things started to not be so great after a while, and that was disappointing. The first situation was when she expressed her concerns about me having little kids. She said that they would always come before her. I instantly thought that this wasn't going to work out. It wasn't fair to her or me. I had a five and two-year-old that were not going anywhere. It would be a long time before they were even grown. I was already struggling with the adjustment not being with them. It was difficult because I cared for her. When she left for work, I packed her things. When she came home, she saw it all by the door and was surprised and upset. She thought about it and understood that they were my children, and they were little kids. I didn't want to waste either of our time. I also understood that my situation was challenging for her as well. She convinced me that she was ok with the situation, and that it was just an adjustment. We made it work for a while.

Money was always tight. I continued to airbrush beeper cases and a lot of them. I was also still exploring painting on paper and canvas with different mediums. I continued my journey to find who I was or going to be as an artist. Still exploring my craft. Art was and still is who I am, and my go to for peace of mind.

One thing Jess and I did not have in common was that she liked to go clubbing and I didn't. I always loved music, but I had too much anxiety to enjoy myself in a room that was full of people, shoulder to shoulder. I have gone in the past, but it was a rare occasion. I'm not one to hold someone back from doing what they want to do though. If she really wanted to go, I wasn't going to stop her. She was her own person, and persistent. She would have me drop her off, so I did. I couldn't take the anxiety and she really loved it. She could handle it; she had gone to clubs alone many times before being with me apparently. She told me she just liked to dance and often saw people there she knew. She was able to go peacefully without me complaining.

One would say I was an asshole; another would say that I was letting her do what she wanted to do. Both are correct, I guess. Now that I think about it, I probably should have gone with her. Maybe I should have sacrificed my mental health to make her happy, or should she have sacrificed going to the club because her boyfriend suffered from crippling anxiety?

So, one day me and Bobby dropped her off at a club in Providence while Bobby and I were driving around in her car, as planned, at her request. She gave me a specific time to pick her up. Shew was only staying for a short time. After I dropped her off, I realize that her car was running out of gas, No cellphones at the time. She's in the club, with our money. I have no money on me, and Bobby doesn't either. It was bad enough that I left her at the club alone. I couldn't leave her there without a ride home. I couldn't communicate with her, so I did what I had to do.

We pulled into a gas station. Many gas stations allowed ya to pump the gas and then pay after. Bobby got out of the car to pump the gas as I stayed in the car ready to take off when we were done. I look in my rearview mirror and he is smoking a blunt as he pumps the gas. I got out of the car and said, "give me that thing before you set yourself on fire". A second after I took the blunt from him, gas backed up and shot into his face. He was seconds away from getting severely burnt. We put a few dollars' worth of gas in the car, we jumped back in, and I floored it. I got just enough gas to pick Jess up from the club and take us all home.

Our landlady was giving us a hard time, so we moved into a new place together. A little bigger, with an extra room for the kids to have a bedroom too. The new apartment was within walking distance from my parents' house. My brother and sister used to come over all the time to visit, which was nice.

They quickly started telling me war stories. I could see the fright in their eyes. They were afraid and didn't want to live with mom anymore. They were persistent that they needed help. I remembered how it was for me before I left home, and it sounded like it had gotten worse for them. The kids were thirteen. My mother was extremely mentally ill, and the more she was treated the worse it seemed to get. I understood what they were saying. I escaped it at seventeen. She couldn't help who she was. It was tough because she was my mother, and my father was caught in the crossfire.

The stories were getting worse, and there was nothing I could do personally. They begged me to help them, and I felt bad. It was a very hard decision to make but I did what I thought was right. The department of child services had already been involved early on, but they were back.

They wanted to live with me, but I was young and kind of a mess emotionally myself. I just couldn't do it and do it right. They ended up going into a foster home together. My brother was removed, and it was the first time they had ever been separated at thirteen years old. I faithfully visited them whenever allowed to. My mother was understandably angry with me. Neither my mother nor father spoke to me for a while. My dad met up with me a couple times, I think that deep down he understood. My mother reported untrue things about me until I was banned from seeing them any longer.

I was having mental health struggles that I didn't even understand yet. Jess was struggling as well with her mental health. One day she slit both wrists in front of me and said, "Look". There were a lot of incidents. I accepted it all and tried to be there for her.

She loved me a lot...for a few days, and then wanted to break up on the next day. It became emotionally exhausting. She would break up and go back, it was back and forth. It seemed like every few days. I didn't want to split up, so I kept going along with what was happening. I was afraid to lose her for good. It became normal, until one time she slept with someone else on the off day. She still wanted to get back with me as she had been doing right along, but it had gone too far that time. History was starting to show that it wasn't going to get any better. I was going to force myself to somehow stay away. Our relationship ended.

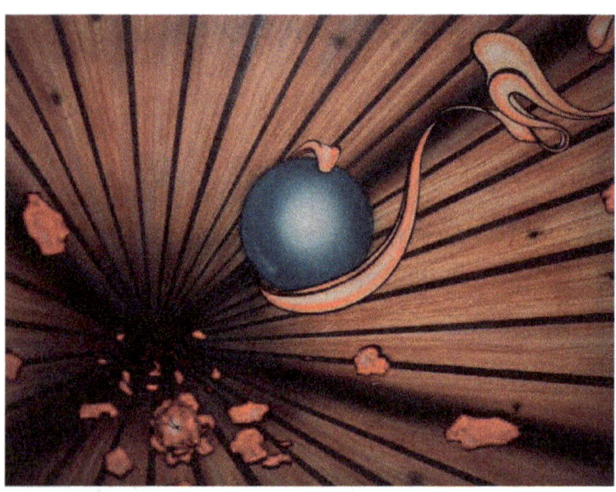

TRANSITON (1998)

This piece opened doors for me to develop myself as an artist.

This acrylic airbrush work is the first painting I made that directed my path towards fine art.

.

Chapter 11

Next Era, My 30s

Besides the airbrushing business, I got another job to help me save up a little extra money to get my own place immediately. I got this little dumpy apartment in Silverlake. Back in the neighborhood I grew up in, except it fell apart and became a shitty area. I could hear rats chewing in the walls at night. I had two windows in my kitchen. I put an air conditioner in each window and right in the middle of them I had a weight bench, instead of a kitchen table. It was the first time in my life that I lived alone. I lifted weights and painted all the time. Friends would be in and out. I was talking to girls. I looked the best I ever had, so it was easy. I needed to occupy my time.

I wasn't looking for a relationship, in fact was trying to avoid it. I was divorced a few years prior and was getting past yet another broken relationship with Jess. I liked her a lot, at least I think I did at the time, everything is relative. I dated several girls before Jess, and She was by far better than any other girl I was with or even dated before her. I talked to a few girls after Jess. Some were cool, and some not so much. I had a lot of experiences in this short time Nothing serious really. I had built up a list of girl's numbers, Some I had dated and some I just hung out with. Some I never met up with.

Jimmy popped back into my life again. He called me up looking for weed. I didn't have any to spare, but I found some for him. It had been a few years, but we started hanging out again instantly. He was an all or nothing kind of person. We were together every day again, but I was a little more aware than in the past. I was conscious that I escaped what could have been an unfortunate situation in the past.

He was a funny guy. One time he showed up at my house and I didn't want to hear it. I was so tired after working all day. I wanted to take a nap. I couldn't keep my eyes open. I don't remember why but there was a pair of big clown glasses and a cowboy hat in the house. He put them on, and he just sat there in the chair beside the bed wearing them, waiting for me to wake up. He was so silly, but he could be rough if triggered. His drug problem had escalated from the earlier days of just having a good time. We always got along well, never argued. I was glad he was back around. He always seemed to be there when I needed him... without asking!

I learned a lot from Jimmy. He taught me how to have a sense of humor. He taught me to be more careless because I worried too much. Although there is a happy medium in that somewhere in between. He also introduced me to drugs a few years back, including hallucinogens. I had a few good times, and some out of body experiences, as well as getting so sick that I thought I was gonna die. Anything more than mushrooms is a bad idea. I was never a big fan of getting fucked up. A little buzz is nice though. I saw enough to know that drugs are bad. I never even really drank much. A little marijuana was always what I liked, it helped with my anxiety, depression, sleeping and my appetite.

Jimmy was also responsible for introducing me to cocaine. It started with me being skeptical and him saying, "Would I ever steer you wrong." A few years prior it was on the dinner plate, until I escaped. Had a few close calls with that too. This time it was only to help me pay my bills and keep a roof over my head. The crappy job I picked up wasn't enough, after losing my business again.

My business with the airbrushed pager cases collapsed after I outsourced a several thousand-piece order for clear coating that came back poorly done. The buyer was displeased and put a stop payment on the check that he had sent me for the order. My business was living week to week, and a hit like that was detrimental.

Jimmy showed me how to buy, cut, bag and sell powder. That didn't last long though. I had too much compassion. Jimmy yelled at me because at times I sent people away. My conscious wouldn't allow me to continue. There is a difference between a good time and when a person knocks on your door every couple of hours all day and night. Ya realize that the person's life is in your hands. Weed was one thing, but I didn't have the heart to enable a person to destroy themselves with real drugs.

I have seen a lot in the drug scene. Enough to keep me clean. Life was very challenging, and no one would have been surprised if I fell in that direction, especially when I was starving for happiness. I saw enough to convince me that drugs were bad. I have seen people's lives fall apart, losing everything including each other. I have seen people die prematurely or go to prison. I saw enough to keep me from going too far. I always knew when it was time to walk away from situations and people. It's not always easy to stand back and look at your life. It's not easy to make changes to alter the path you're on, but I did!

I had no goals or plans, I just wanted to get by and be happy. My list of lady friends was getting long, I was just having fun. As always trying to make light of any challenges and create a life that was worth living. I always looked young for my age, and I've always been young hearted. No one believed that I was only twenty-seven. People made a big deal over it, often asking to see my ID, and it became annoying. To make my life easy I started saying I was twenty-five. It was easier to believe I suppose. It didn't matter because I was just trying to occupy my time, nothing serious. I was having innocent fun. Making the best out of life, as always. Besides that, I continued to paint.

I spent a lot of time alone in my dumpy apartment listening to rats scurrying through the walls. I'd blast music to drown out the noise. I'd roll a few blunts and take off all my clothes. I was alone and free. I'd paint for hours. I didn't mind living alone for a little while, but sometimes it got a little creepy. It wasn't the best neighborhood either. I painted a few murals on the walls in that apartment to try and make it look better. It was an experience.

I got a new job at an auto parts store that was paying better, a new place to live while I pulled my life back together a little. I was at work one day and this girl walked in and was buying air fresheners or something like that for her car. All I saw was the back of her. Not many girls came in the store, so she stood out. I didn't pay her much mind other than that, until I saw her again a few days later. I was walking into work and noticed her for a second time, and she had a nice car. I said, "Nice car". She came in and bought some more stuff it. I was at work, so I had to be discreet, and I wrote my number on her receipt.

Her name was Katrina. She called me the next night; we talked a little bit and planned a date. That weekend we went out. At that time, we were both partyers. I started seeing her more, because we had a good time. Katrina became someone that I saw more and more. We liked each other but were not official. She was reluctant and wanted to take it slow after leaving a prior bad relationship. That was a good Idea, since I also had just left a relationship recently before that. She questioned my income and was embarrassed by the car I drove. She was a little shallow, but I didn't care, I was just having fun. We started to spend more time together, mainly as friends that might be taking it further.

It was healthy to live alone for a while, until it wasn't. I came home from work one day and opened the front door of the apartment. I looked down at the floor and saw a music CD lying there. I thought to myself that I have that same CD. Thinking the people on the first floor must have it too and dropped it. I stepped over it and continued to walk up the stairs until I saw a second CD, that I also owned. I walked up those stairs faster and cringed as I turned the corner on that last step leading to my apartment. I looked up at my door with fright and my door was swinging wide open.

I walked in my place and the first thing I noticed was that my TV and stereo were gone. I paid a thousand dollars for that thing. I made weekly payments at a furniture rental place until it was paid off and it was gone. My dresser was pulled out where my rent money was hidden underneath it. Even my jar of change was gone. Even the little bit of weed I had left was gone. I couldn't even smoke my sorrows away that day.

I thought it was the kid that used to work at my store because he had picked up a nasty drug habit. Not all my furniture was pulled out, just the one dresser that I kept my rent money under, and he knew that. I went to his house and barged in. I grabbed him and hung him out the second- floor window. Then I thought it out, it cost me a lot, but I just got this kid out of my life for good. He was a person from my old life left over, and he lingered. Once a friend, he brought negative energy that I didn't need.

My friend Ricky was going to college for the winter semester and going four ways on a nice one-family cottage in Bonnet shore, down by the water in South County. They only had three people and needed a fourth. So, I went for it. At this point, I had nothing to lose. It was only for the winter, so I only had a few months. It was a fun time. There were a few keg parties there, but they were drug free.

I got a warehouse job that paid a lot more than I was making at the auto parts store. I applied and got that job, and I then got a second job at UPS. I was unloading trucks all morning and loading them at night. I never worked so hard in my life.

Katrina wasn't getting along with her mother and wanted to move out of her house. She was nineteen but appeared to be much older. In fact, I thought she was about twenty-five when I first met her. I was shocked when I found out how old she was, I almost didn't date her.

She was making plans to go live with her friend Missy who had an escalating drug problem. Missy was robbing work to support a two hundred dollar a day drug habit, and that's 90's money. Being an addict was right around the corner for Katrina too, from what I could tell. Jimmy was heading in the same direction. I felt like I had the power to make a difference in her life.

At that point I cared about Katrina's wellbeing, and I had a bad feeling about it. I felt that Katrina was impressionable, and I knew it would have a bad ending for her if she went to live with her. Missy was a female version of Jimmy but in overdrive. I was afraid to make that move but I did it for Katrina. We agreed nothing would change, she would live her life and I would live mine. We would get back together at the end of the day. I made a decision that was about to be life changing. Katrina moved in with me down in Bonnet Shore. We partied a lot and had a good time.

Within a very short time her grandmother, who was basically like a parent to her unexpectedly died. Things became very hard for us from day one. She was heartbroken, I felt bad. The honeymoon period ended very fast, if there was one at all. She was going through a lot at the time. I was dealing with Rhonda, who was giving me a hard time, we weren't getting along. Katrina and I were more friendly than romantic from the start. We just started dating and were immediately living together. We didn't truly know each other yet. She was suffering from a loss. We stopped partying, I put an end to that. It wasn't a healthy lifestyle. I told her that I wanted to live a clean life and she agreed.

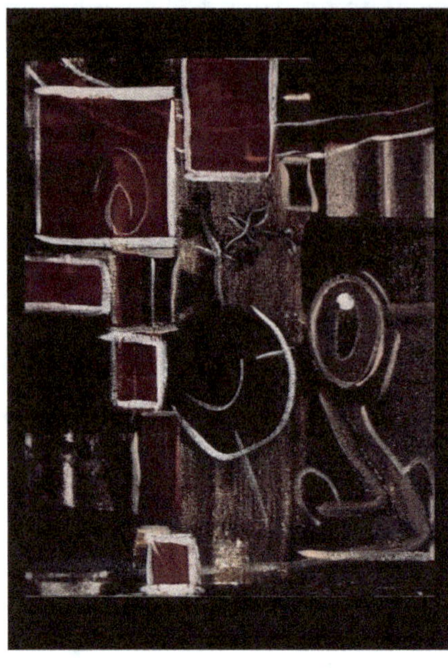

KNOWLEDGE
(1999)

This acrylic painting displays my transition from airbrushing on paper to using a bristle brush on canvas.

After missing out on much of my childhood, especially my teenage years, I found myself learning and absorbing as much knowledge as possible as a young adult... Learning how to be human.

The winter season ended, and it was time to move out of Bonnet Shore. We moved into Katrina's grandmother's empty apartment. Her mom and fourteen-year-old sister Judy lived next door. Katrina's father was older and became sick at an early age. I was the first man living in this house in many years. I certainly had my work cut out for me. I struggled to make the house as nice as I could. Learning as I went along. I was getting older, approaching my thirties. I was hustling day and night. We both worked, and I had two jobs. I also registered for Art classes at a local college.

Shortly after, Missy, the girl Katrina almost moved in with was found dead in a crack house. I truly believe that if I hadn't entered Katrina's life, she would have been dead as well. I truly believe that I saved her life, one hundred percent. The relationship also gave me a more constructive life.

Chapter 12

Exploring My Artistic Direction

I was trying to pull my life together. I felt like I was always trying to pull my life together. Art remained an important part of my life and I experimented with different art mediums and techniques. I started painting just canvases, with acrylic paints. I was edging towards fine art. I decided that I wanted to show my work to a gallery for some feedback.

I knew nothing about the business at all. I had a pile of paintings. It was a mixture of all different styles, and different techniques. I opened the phone book and picked a random gallery. I had no idea what I was doing. I was learning and teaching myself about art, how to make art, what art was, and the business around it.

I found a gallery. One of the nicest galleries in Providence, with this sweet old lady curating it. I was putting myself out there. I knew I was swimming in dangerous waters. Art was beginning to be even more important to me than ever before. If she trashed me, I was liable to never paint again.

The art business is rough. You can tell her gallery was sophisticated, and she was classy. Her gallery was elegant and beautiful, and the artwork hanging up was amazing. I quickly realized that I was way out of my league being there. This lady was direct and firm. I thought that I was about to be torn down. She had been dealing in art her whole life. I didn't belong there.

I was there though, and I was doing it. She said, "Show me what you have". I placed each piece I had on her table. She was the first person that had ever seen my work. She said, "Well, you definitely have talent." This is the kind of lady that would have told me if I shouldn't be painting at all. Then she said, "I can tell that you're still learning, find yourself and what you want to paint". She was right, but I needed that direction from someone that knew art. I will never forget her, she was very inspiring and made me feel like I had potential, and that I wasn't crazy. I actually had real talent.

I had many styles going on. I was raw, and inexperienced and all over the place. She was right, I was learning. Visiting her was part of my process. Serious art is something that takes time to develop. As I grew, I truly learned to understand this. It's been many years now. Recently I looked her up because I wanted to show her how far I've come. I came to learn that she passed away a few years ago at the age of ninety-four. God Bless her soul. She is one of many major influences and motivators that I have been privileged to meet who still to this day encourages my creativity. The drive to truly succeed. . As I started my journey as an artist, I continued to struggle trying to fix Katrina's crumbling house. The roof was leaking. The plumbing and electrical were bad. I was disguising it with nice landscaping. I did a lot, and I was getting overwhelmed. I was doing it all myself. I was no carpenter, but I was ambitious. It seemed like a fresh start. Katrina and I both needed to heal and live a better life than we had been.

Jimmy was gone and then was back around again. He would come and go like that sometimes. This time he had a landscaping business, and I hired him. He spent a couple days there. It looked great when he was done. I missed Jimmy's friendship, but he was always unstable. He had already spent some time in prison. Many of his friends were dying around him. We talked a little. He looked rough. He used to always be clean cut; the ladies always liked him. It was obvious that he was challenging life hard. I had a feeling that it was the last time that I would ever see him.

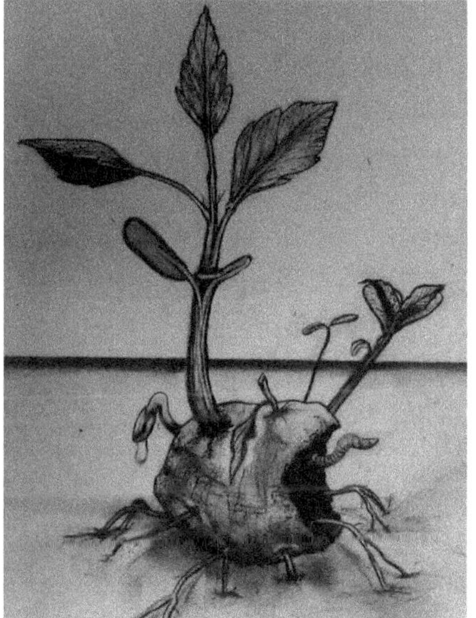

REBIRTH- Charcoal on paper (2009)

Katrina and I were fighting a lot, we had been since day one. It became the way it was after a while. From my point of view, she was very aggressive. She could be outright mean when something upset her, and it didn't take much. It seemed to me that she had an anger management problem. At one point she was grabbing my paintings off the wall and throwing them at me. She simply couldn't control herself. She would burst with hatred. Some paintings would be thrown from the second floor. Usually missed me, but a few made contact.

I went to work and came home. I had a few little hobbies and was a family man. For some reason I made her angry a lot. She ruined my things, threw stuff and hit me often. My self-esteem was starting to deteriorate. I don't think she ever really liked me much. I believe the relationship was just convenient for her. It was hard to ever truly make her happy. Eventually I think I stopped trying so hard.

I have one painting that was unintentionally completed by her. It was thrown across the room at me. The impact it made from hitting the floor created diagonal cracks in the paint. The painting was very important to me and my father. I couldn't disregard it. Fortunately, the cracks were even, and they resembled rain falling on a dark rainy day. Perfect for the meaning and events of this particular piece of artwork. It was the last painting that my father saw. The painting was a top view of the house I was raised in, in Silver Lake. It's a dark painting, with leaves falling from the tree in a storm. With real leaves painted on and applied to the painting.

Mostly from misdirected anger, I endured a lot. It changed me as a person. I think she was angry with herself and the choices she had made in life. I came home from work on more than one occasion to photos with me in them ripped up into pieces. This one time I came home, and she was with her sister trying to scrub marker scribbles off my paintings. I don't know why I went through that, but I think it's because I had low self-esteem. I didn't think much of myself. I was very insecure. Growing up I saw my mother treat my father poorly. So, it wasn't unusual to me, although I hoped that it would stop one day.

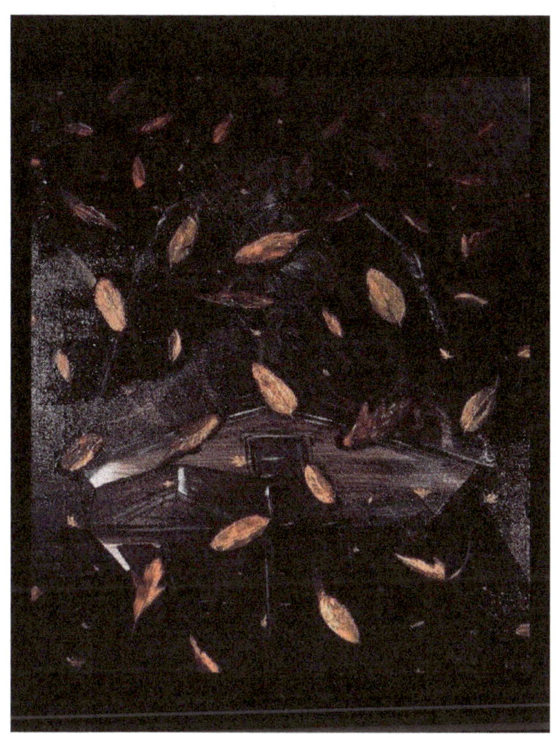

STORM
(2001)

This mixed media composition was the last painting that my father saw me create. It is of the home I grew up in, on a windy autumn day. Later the cracks added gave it the appearance of falling rain, a fiercer storm.

Chapter 13

Emotional Devastation

With all the challenges, finally some good news for a change. My mother was going to take my brother back home from the group home that he had been staying in. He was so excited, and I drove over to go visit him. When I pulled up to the house, I saw that he was sitting on the front stairs and seemed upset. He looked at me and said, "She changed her mind". He was so sad, and I felt bad for him. I ended up taking him in with me. You rarely see it when you are in it but looking back it's clear that I was in over my head myself, but I was gonna give it my best shot.

I gave him as good of an environment as I could. He tested the limits a couple times like any teenager, but he was genuinely a good kid. I just didn't want to see him suffer anymore. He had been pushed from group home to foster home to group home. It was a vicious cycle. I know he was in pain from our mother's rejection. I couldn't allow him to go through this any longer.

My sister was lucky enough to not be moved around as

often. The word lucky is used lightly. She was anything but lucky. Her situation sucked as well. The whole thing sucked. To this day I feel guilty for not taking them in when they were thirteen. I know I wasn't equipped to care for them well, but at least they would have been loved. Theres no way of always knowing the right answers. Realizing mistakes when it's too late to recover from it.

They are more to me than just siblings. I was there when they were born and took care of them when there was no one else capable, or available. We all experienced the same situation, but from a different angle. We all have a special bond, at least, I think so. I love them both very much. I hope they understand and forgive me.

I have always relied on my artwork to feel better, creating art has always kept me whole. I would more than often paint late at night. It was peaceful, and no one was awake to bother me. Once everyone was sleeping for the night I'd head to my basement where I kept an art studio. I buried myself in the room and painted for hours and hours. Experimenting like a scientist in my laboratory. I'd have work in the morning too, but it didn't matter. Work was what I did to pay the bills, being an Artist was what I was.

I was full of energy and able to function just fine on a couple hours of sleep. I did that for a while. I had a lot of alone time in the middle of the night. I had a lot of time to think, maybe sometimes too much time. I created a lot of artworks during that time.

So much time had passed. So many things had happened, including 911. It was a scary, yet a united time. For the first time in my life, Americans' felt vulnerable. We were in shock. There have been so many changes. Art is one thing that has always been present in my life through everything. As I documented my own life and emotions.

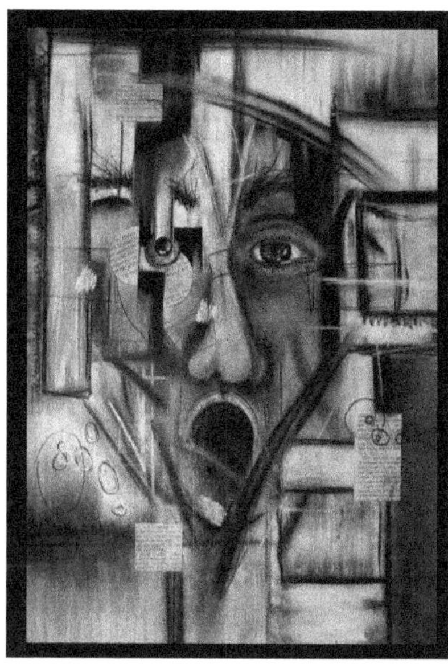

SHOCK

(2001)

This charcoal on paper drawing was created the week following the 911 attack on America.

Always moving in a forward direction. Probably the only thing I was good at, just being me. My love of creating things never changed. Even though I was rarely ever satisfied with what I made, it's still what I am best at. Every mistake was a lesson learned, making me one step closer to my goal. That is what kept me motivated, and still does. I believed in myself, and I was confident that I would one day be successful. God helps those who help themselves. The path to every goal is a scrambled puzzle that needs to be strategically put together.

My brother and I had become close like we were when he was a little kid, when I left him on that floor coloring many years before. We were both adults and became friends. We were hanging out this one night like we usually did. I just finished smoking a blunt, and the phone rang. It was my aunt, and I couldn't make out what she was saying. She was crying in hysterics. The only thing I could make out is when she said the words, "Your father". In the middle of all her crying.

I knew immediately something bad happened to him. Finally, she got her words out. My father was in the ambulance, and they were trying to bring him back to life. I dropped to my knees and bawled my eyes out. I knew my father was gone. Katrina took my keys to work with her by mistake that day, so I had no way of getting to the hospital. That probably happened for a reason. I was in no condition to drive at that moment. There was no ride share then, and all the taxis were backed up for over an hour. Finally, I reached my friend Ricky who picked me up and took me to the hospital.

I will never forget arriving at the hospital, and that long elevator ride up. Walking down the hall to the room in the hospital seemed to take so long, peeking in each room as I walked by them, thinking it could be him. Then finally reaching the right room. I saw my father's lifeless body lying on the table.

Doctors and nurses were all working on him. He had a tube sticking out of an incision they made in his chest. Wires and machines and people everywhere. It was so frightening to know that my father's life was on the edge of death. He was breathing again, but he was nonresponsive. I saw his eyes open, and his fingers twitch. I got so excited thinking he was waking up, then the nurse told me that those were involuntary movements. It was such a dark moment.

They didn't know if he was brain dead or not. He was possibly without oxygen for forty-five minutes or more. My mother looked at me and told me that it was my fault if he died. She elaborated saying I should have been more helpful.

They had just recently moved. I was in school and working full time. I was trying, but. I guess I didn't try hard enough. He moved the small stuff alone on a day that I wasn't available. A moving company moved the heavy stuff. I was full of even more guilt that I would carry a lifetime.

He had a small heart attack a few years back, and I was in denial that his heart wasn't at its best. I acted like it didn't happen. The thought of losing him was horrifying. He always said that he would live to be ninety and I believe him. He was strong, mentally and physically. Plus, he was only in his sixties.

The EMT guys were able to bring Dad back to life in the ambulance right after he dropped to the ground in front of my aunt's house. It took my aunt a few minutes to realize that he was lying on the ground. My mother was hugging him saying goodbye, never calling for help. Neither of them acted fast enough. I resented my mother for a long time for not acting faster. I later understood more that in that moment she was sure he was dead. She wanted those few last moments with him alone. My mother figured that was her chance to say bye for the last time, versus maybe we can save him, I guess. I think her life flashed before her, as though it was her own death in that moment.

My father had been in the hospital for a little over a week and I was going to visit him every day. Talking to him in case he could hear me. Checking on him and discussing tests performed with the doctors. The big question was if he was ever going to wake up and how much of his brain was destroyed due to the lack of oxygen.

Katrina was getting frustrated and annoyed with it all. I

believe she felt as though I was spending too much time at the hospital. The normal flow of life had been interrupted. It was becoming an inconvenience to her life I suppose. One day she looked at me and said, "What are you waiting for?". Meaning, I was taking too long making the final decision on removing life support from my father. At this point machines were assisting him. How much we weren't sure yet.

I needed to feel confident that there was no hope, before I gave up on him. I was his advocate. His breathing another day was solely depending on me. At the time I wanted the hospital to test everything they could. I needed to make sure there wasn't any possibility of him waking up before I was able to let him go. It seemed to me that Katrina was rushing me, making me believe that I needed to just let him die. I'm sure it was inconvenient, but it was my dad that raised me. I needed to do what I needed to do. He was what was important at that time.

She damaged our relationship, creating a wound that I would learn to realize would never heal. After that it was just me hanging on. I was a lost soul. On the day of the funeral my son Jr saw his first dead person, his grandfather. I have the vision of my father lying in the casket burnt into my memory.

I remember sitting in the limousine and looking back at the church, I saw my father standing there watching his own funeral. Maybe I was delusional, or maybe it was real. I'll always believe in my heart that his spirit was there. Observing us mourn his passing and celebrating his life. My mother was a mess, so wasn't I. She told me that my father was disappointed in me. The idea that my father died thinking little of me hurt so bad. I'll take that pain to my grave.

After my father died, I went to his grave and just sat there for hours, even bringing lunch and a blanket. I was taking it badly and dealing with it alone. I had guilt weighing heavy on my shoulders. My mother placed blame on me. The last time I saw him he asked me to come over and see the new place they had just moved into. He was excited to show me the pond on the property that had ducks in it. Like the ducks we used to go to feed many years back. I was too busy with work and school, so I didn't make it over. Talk about regret!

Man, I wish I had a do over for that day. I remember turning the corner and looking back at him for the last time as though I knew it was the last time deep down inside. I had an empty feeling. I should have followed my instinct, made the sacrifice and went to see him. I feel guilty about that.
I spent a year slowly drawing a picture of Jesus. It was my way of dealing with the pain of losing him, and the guilt that I now had overpowering my soul. That picture I drew is how I visualize the Prayer Our Father, in my head. Jesus is in heaven with flowers pouring from his hands onto the earth. Making it on earth as it is in heaven, peaceful and beautiful. I used charcoal with a slight pastel accent. I sat alone late at night with my thoughts. I did a little bit every day. It was my therapy.

My parents lived in East Providence. They lived in an apartment building together with their two Siamese cats for just a few weeks. Apartment nine eleven, go figure. It's funny how life works sometimes. My father moved them into a place that she was able to somewhat manage alone. Just a few weeks prior they were living in a situation that she would never have been able to maintain.

There was a cemetery right next door from their new place. My father was buried in that cemetery. My mother spent a lot of time there at the grave as I did. One time I went there, and it looked as though someone was digging in the dirt. I questioned my mother, and she told me that she was trying to dig him up. She wanted to be with him again. She was digging with her bare hands. Saying that neither of us were taking it well would have been an understatement, and I don't think anyone realized how bad it had become.

I spent much of my days off from work and many nights after work with my mother. I spent a lot of time with her at first, she wasn't used to being alone. I had to teach her how to manage life. She was totally dependent on my father for over thirty years, and she was severely mentally ill. She didn't even know how to pay her bills. She asked to move in with me, but I was afraid to do it. I was afraid it would affect my mental health, and history told me that Katrina wouldn't like it. I didn't want to upset her; it didn't take much. Life was already very hard to manage. I wish I could have done more for my mother than I did. If it were now, I would have moved her in with me.

Shortly after my mother had a friend, a boyfriend. I caught this man wearing my father's clothes one day. He was younger, and I had words with him a few times, because I was just angry, and it was too soon. He had some brain damage from a car accident, and it was like talking to a child. He also lived in the same building as my mother. It was extremely upsetting, my father was barely cold, and she was devastated over his death. I was very confused and angry.

When the dust settled a little and I had a clearer head, I realized that she was afraid of being alone. She had me but obviously I was not her partner. She was always planning on how she was going to get by financially and even more, emotionally. Her new friend had nothing to do with her love for my father. She kept an eight by ten photo of my father on her dresser. She talked about him all the time and she was deteriorating slowly. She was still in survival mode from her childhood.

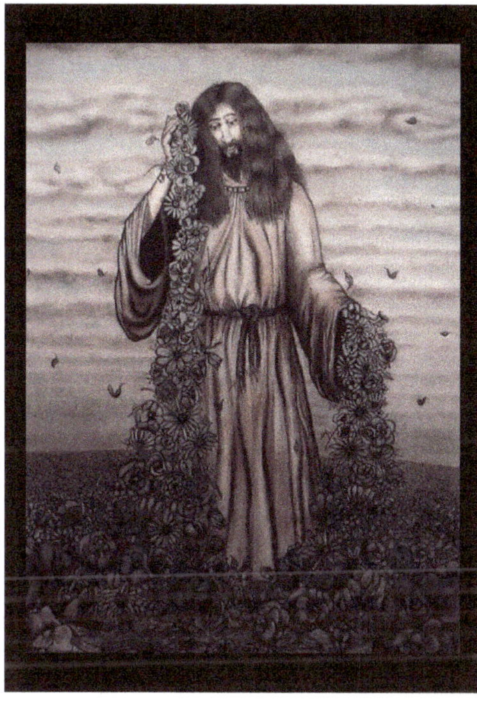

FATHER

(2001)

This Charcoal on paper drawing was created slowly over the twelve months following my father's death.

I was juggling caring for my mother who was nearly helpless and managing a relationship with Katrina that had been damaged. I still hadn't been allowed the proper time to do my own mourning. It was my father that I loved so much, that had died suddenly, and I was expected to be the strong one. I ultimately dropped out of college. My mind was in a bad place, and not feeling well emotionally, and still silently angry with Katrina for rushing me, and then not being there for me emotionally in the way I needed her to.

My dad had a small heart attack a few years before he died, and I was in denial that his heart wasn't at its best. I acted like it didn't happen after. The thought of losing him was horrifying. He always said that he would live to be ninety and I believed him. He was strong, mentally and physically. Plus, he was only in his sixties. He appeared to be healthy.

I was bitter with Katrina. I recalled this one of many times that I called my dad when he was alive. Asking him to pick me up because Katrina was fighting with me. This one time he said to me, "Don't be like me, and live your life like that". I ended up leaving Katrina shortly after. We weren't married, and we didn't have any kids. I was disgusted with her, and we split up.

The only apartment I could afford was ironically on the next street over from where my parents lived off Atwells Ave., right before they moved, and my father died. The house was such a dump and had roaches. My Buddy Josh and I had been hanging out again for a while as adults and helped me move in on a hot summer day. It must have been 90 degrees and humid. It was just me and my little brother living there. It had only been a few weeks, but I needed to feel better. I was young and quickly learned that there were girls that would treat me much better than Katrina did.

It had only been a few weeks and I went by Katrina's one morning to get something, if I remember correctly. When I arrived, there was a different car in the driveway. It was a supped up little sports car. It was obviously another guy's car and he obviously slept over, in a bed that was mine weeks prior. The dating part... I understood, wanting to move on. It was him in the same house that I had lived in with her for three years just weeks after was the part that I didn't understand, especially if she didn't want to break up as she said. The same house that I invested my time, energy and money into that I didn't even own. This guy mind as well have been wearing my clothes.

I was young and my ego was too big for my own good, or maybe it was the roaches in my new apartment, or maybe because it was on the next street over from my parents' old place. The same house I ran away from twelve years earlier. Either way, I decided to talk to her. I rang the doorbell and then threw pebbles at her window when she didn't answer the door. She came outside and discussed trying again. To get back together she gave me ultimatums. She said the only way we would get back together is if we got married and had a baby. She said she would change her ways, and I believed her. So, we got married a couple of weeks after.

I can remember starting second guessing the relationship quickly after. Her true colors shined bright once again quickly once she was pregnant. When she became angry, she would tell me that she was carrying another man's baby. This happened countless times and it was such a mind fuck. Because she was just with another guy, so it was possible. I started to wonder sometimes if she was maybe telling the truth when she said that. It was a mind fuck to say the least.

She would often like to open the phone book in front of me. Antagonizing me as she looked for an abortion clinic. She was doing it just to freak me out, I think. She knew I had mental health issues of some sort, so it wasn't difficult to turn me into a ball of anxiety. I was an easy emotional target. It was her way of hurting me, and it worked.

It just added to the trauma I already had stored up inside me. I was telling myself I couldn't do it, because she was pregnant with my child. So, I gave the relationship my best. It was not easy. The hard feelings were deeper than I had originally thought. I realized that things would probably never be the same between us again.

The gynecologist called a few weeks before Christmas and told us that the baby showed signs of possibly having down syndrome. We were given the choice of ending the pregnancy if we wanted to, and we declined. That was the first and only Christmas in my life that I didn't have a Christmas tree. The next few months were worrisome. Hoping the baby was going to be ok.

Chapter 14

Purpose

I remember the day my daughter was born. She was two weeks early. The delivery was difficult. The baby was having a hard time delivering. They were about to use a vacuum until Katrina vomited. Her muscles contracted from vomiting, pushing the baby right out. My baby was a girl. She was beautiful. Quickly I realized that she was not breathing. There was a lot of commotion, and it was very scary. She finally cried and took her first breath. She was ok. She also was not a down syndrome baby.

I couldn't hold her for a little bit, she was wearing a tiny oxygen mask, crying and crying. I just kept staring at her and taking pictures. It was a moment I'll never forget. Her crying was the most beautiful sound I had ever heard. I started crying myself from emotion. In an instant I had a purpose and a reason to be my best. Holding her for the first time was an amazing feeling. When I woke up in the morning I couldn't wait to get her from the nursery in the morning. Taking her home and taking care of her is all I wanted to do.
I was thirty years old, a grown man. Becoming a father as an adult was different than becoming a father when you are a

kid yourself having kids. I was more mature when she was born and ready to be a dad. The best was leaving the hospital; with her. I had so much heartache before that. Just a year prior, I lost my father, and I was lost. I had this void in my life, and my new baby daughter filled it. She gave me purpose again. A fresh start to life. A new beginning.

I would wake up for the nighttime feedings, even after I returned to work. I fixed up her bedroom really nice, it was the nicest room in the house. I enjoyed taking care of my daughter. Just a few weeks later she was baptized. My old friend Josh became her godfather. He was good to her, I must say. Life was coming together, now that I had my daughter. I had another shot at having a family. It appeared that the pieces were coming together once again.

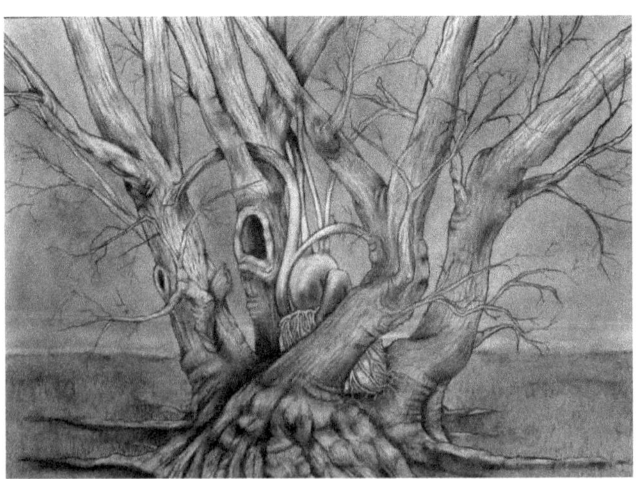

TREE OF LIFE (2011)
Drawing of a tree with a heart in the center.
Charcoal on paper.

I was a good provider. I am an artist, but I've worked jobs in retail management to pay the bills for most of my adult life. Retail Management was never the right job for me, but I was good at it. The key is treating the people under you like people. Be their leader and not their boss. But sales means being pushy, and a manager means being bossy. Neither of those qualities are who I am. I just had to bullshit my way through. It wasn't me, but I knew what needed to be done. Earning and providing for myself and those that depend on me was most important at that time. Growing up in a financially challenged home caused me to be petrified of poverty my entire life.

Although a void was filled with my daughter's birth, I still had a hard time dealing with my father's death, I went to therapy and took anti-depressants. My new baby daughter gave me something to fight for. I really wish my father got to meet her; he would have adored her too. It was nice that my mother got to see her. It's too bad that she was too out of it to really be able to enjoy her granddaughter, like a grandmother should.

At six months old my daughter gave me yet another scare. It was the first time that she had spiked a high fever. It was just her and I that day. She was lethargic, and I was getting very nervous. I took her to the nearby children's hospital ER in Providence. Katrina met us there. The hospital staff ran a bunch of tests and couldn't find a reason for her fever. The bad news was that one test had shown fluid around her brain. I had never been so scared in my life. They said there was a chance that my six-month-old daughter might have meningitis. This could become deadly if not treated.

I was in shock for a minute. I asked all the what-if questions. The only way to know for sure was drawing fluid from her spine. Of course, we didn't want to do this. The alternative was that we took her home and she would either not have meningitis, or she would die from meningitis.

It was not a risk that I was willing to take. I stood in the parking lot crying. I recall the moment I first saw her when they were finished. She was silent with no emotion. She was obviously traumatized. She was just staring straight ahead. In her baby mind, she went through something confusing and painful, and I was not there to protect her. I can't help but think that night caused her some permanent emotional trauma that followed her throughout life.

We adults understand it was to be sure she was safe, but she was a baby. All she knew was that the people she trusted left her alone with people who hurt her. Every experience we go through in life, good or bad, makes us who we are.

The good news was that she did not have meningitis. The following day we went to her pediatrician where she was examined again. The diagnosis was that she simply had an ear infection. The hospital claimed to not see it during the examination, so they said. I then learned that there is nothing the hospital can do for a fever that can't be done at home. That was a scary night, but I am grateful she was ok.

Katrina's mom was excited to have a granddaughter. She was a sweet ol' lady. We have lived next door to each other for a few years. She was as helpful as she could be. My mother would come over occasionally, on weekends. I have a precious picture of her pushing my daughter on the swing. I was happy that she got to have two grandmothers. I never had even one.

Unfortunately, Katrina's mom became terminally ill during this time. It seemed to be getting progressively worse. It was so sad when I heard that one of her wishes was to live long enough to see my daughter walk. She was not really that old, but sickness made her old. She was no longer able to work and had little money coming in. For good reasons, she was having serious financial challenges. The poor lady was being harassed by creditors daily, and they had no sympathy. The house became too much for her to handle. This was my chance to do what I could for her. She was in need, I had resources.

Right before my daughter was born, I started that new job at a Cell Phone store and within a year I was promoted to manager. I hated it, but I was pretty good at it. It just was not who I was, an artist. It was a good job though and it certainly paid the bills. Things became a little easier financially. I was working hard while hanging on to the aspiration of being a successful artist.

I became the primary bread winner in this house. Buying the house was presented to me by Katrina. I made the decision to buy it from her mom. It was also projected to be good for us in the long run as well. It was an old and ugly house. I didn't get a deal, that wasn't the purpose of this transaction. We Purchased it for more than was owed. It gave her mother some money to put in her pocket so she could enjoy life a little more before she passed. Plus, Katrina and her sister were able to stay in the house they grew up in for a while longer. Up until then our rent was low. Katrina's mom did not have a mortgage, just taxes and insurance. We were now paying a full mortgage, but never charged her mom anything for rent.

Life was a hustle. Working this mentally exhausting job, doing my best to be a husband and a good dad. Like most families it became a vicious cycle of trying to pay the bills. There were some good times, especially with my baby girl. My world revolved around her. Katrina was still difficult to get along with. She was more than often angry. There were a lot of times that were just tolerable. I wanted to make life changes countless times over the years but couldn't do it. I needed to wait for my daughter to be old enough. Unfortunately, I think Katrina had a mean streak in her and she would have done all she could to destroy me and the relationship my daughter had with me.

I loved my daughter to death, and I wouldn't trade her for anything. So, if that meant I had to sacrifice to stay in her life raising her, then I was going to, and I did. She filled the empty hole in my heart that was left when my father died. She was thought to maybe have Down Syndrome before she was even born. She wasn't breathing at birth. Spinal tap at six months old. She was brand new and already facing so many challenges. I was not leaving her side.

She was and still is a blessing. I spent as much time as I could with her as she grew up. As far as I could see her mom was not as much of a nurturer as I was, so I felt as though I had to play the role of a dad-mom. Doing that, I was accused of coddling her. I was just trying to give her the love and special care that knew she needed at the time. I know her mother loved her, but in my opinion, she didn't love having a child like I did. My daughter always knew that I was there for her.

I really enjoyed raising her. We would sit on the floor and play. More than often, we would draw and color together. She drew very well and had a great imagination as early as just a few years old. It was impressive. She later started to write stories. She didn't stick with it as I wished she did, but her destiny is hers to fulfil. Maybe one day she will. I saved many of her work and still have them to this day.

She was challenging at times, but I put in the hard work needed. In my opinion, I was the only one that truly understood her. I believe we always had a bond, especially when she was little. She unfortunately clashed with her mother a lot. I believe they had similar personalities and they seemed to have no patience for each other at times.

My son was getting older and like most kids, he started to act out. I caught him smoking weed in front of the laundry mat on Cranston Street one day. I pulled over and said, "Get in". I drove him to the roughest neighborhood I could find. He said, "What are you doing?" I told him, "I'm just dropping you off to hang out and make new friends." He said, "What do you mean dropping me off"? I said, "Get out of the car and make some friends." Then he said, "Alright I get it." I tried to guide him in the right direction. It's not easy when your kid doesn't live with you.

I knew there were issues starting up with him in his mom's house. He wasn't getting along with Jack. He was fourteen years old, right at the age where kids start testing the waters to see how much they can get away with. It was time that he was with his father. I wanted to raise him from day one. Unfortunately, it wasn't an option.

Tammy was only two when her mother and I divorced, and Jack has been there ever since. Of course, I hated Jack in the beginning, but now that I look back, at least Rhonda picked a person who grew up to be a decent guy. He was good to my kids, as far as I am aware of. But I missed out on a lot because of him, so didn't the kids. But it is what it is, and Jack was a kid himself at that time. So, I don't hold it against him so much anymore. I hate that I was often judged for not being around more, even though I was around and always present. I was never gone. A few years prior my kids were taken from me and raised by a teenager. It really fucked me up bad. I do not think anyone realized how badly that affected me. I was doing my best to be my best. Even when it wasn't great. I was struggling.

My son Jr called me frantic one day. He had been acting up a little. His mom's boyfriend was having a tough time dealing with it and it was escalating. As I heard it, they both started to get handsy with each other. I knew that they had not been getting along. Rhonda and I were quite different people, so we did not get along well. She constantly gave me a hard time, which made co-parenting difficult. She was allowing her boyfriend to handle situations that he clearly needed help with. I think he was sincerely trying. She was too but didn't handle things in the best ways possible. I'm speculating, I wasn't in their house. Either way, it was not working out, and my son was at a vulnerable age.

I am sure my son was giving him a hard time; he was a teenager. My son needed to be with me, his father. They got into a physical altercation and enough was enough. I got in my car and flew over there as fast as I could. I pulled up, parked in the middle of the street. I yelled out, "Where's my fucking son." I said, "Get him and make sure he brings his clothes with him". Nobody said a word to me, they just let it happen. I probably could have and should have handled it a little better, but it was my son, and it brought out a little aggression from me. My son got in the car and that was it. I took him home to live with me.

It was nice having my son with me. I waited ten years to have him back in my life full-time again. The first thing we did was start a project together. We remodeled the hallway leading into the basement, where we built him a bedroom. Two exits and fire-retardant drywall. I made sure he was safe. He had his own space with privacy, something he was not used to. Right next door to his bedroom I built my art studio. Before that I was painting in what was an old dirty basement. Now I had my son back again and a nice clean place to do my artwork. I was happy about that.

We were able to open the doors between his room and my art studio, both rooms we built together. We spent a lot of quality time together. I taught him how to airbrush. He loved art too. We are only nineteen years apart, so we listened to the same music and could really enjoy a good conversation.

I came home this one time from work and saw a bunch of police cars at the bottom of my street. They had their guns drawn. I was filled with anxiety; this was happening a couple hundred feet from my front door. There were two people in the middle of the street, on their knees with their hands behind their heads. I got a little closer and I saw that one of these people was my son. I jumped out of my car and ran towards him, with no regard for the guns drawn. The police screamed at me and quickly got me out of there. Watching the police car drive off with my son in the back seat was heart breaking. As the police car drove off, he looked at me out the back window. The look of sadness on his face is burnt into my memories forever.

That unfortunately was not the last legal situation. I've had my house searched by the police. He even did a little time in the boy's correction facility for assault, even though he was just protecting a friend from a bully. He made the mistake of taking the kids' phone after knocking him out, just to be a punk. He turned that assault charge into a robbery charge. I will never forget going to court for his arraignment. They walked him in wearing handcuffs. On his way out I walked up to him and gave him a hug and whispered in his ear. I told him I had a friend of a friend that was gonna keep an eye on him on the inside. He whispered back in my ear, "It's not bad there, don't worry." Although I was relieved that he felt safe, it was alarming. If he had no fear, then he learned nothing, and I feared that he would repeat.

I became harder on him, I needed to be. He challenged the fuck out of me. My son had no idea how much I loved him and still do. Growing up, his mom was a little too easy on him, jack was limited because he isn't his dad. I was limited because he didn't live with me, but then I had him full time. I did my best to make the best impression on him that I could in the short time he had as a teenager.

He was about seventeen and started not coming home for days at a time. I became frustrated because we had already discussed this several times. One night I told him to come home that night or not to come back at all. I was surprised when he picked not to come home at all. That was not how I expected it to go. He started couch hopping and never came back. I didn't see him for a while after that. Another heartbreaking moment.

It appeared that he became out of control when he came to live with me. Of course, I was judged for that. The fact is that I happened to have him during the roughest of his teenage years. I like to think I was influential in his life at that crucial time. He told me many years later that if it weren't for my parenting during that time, the trouble he got into would have been ten times worse.

My son had always chosen a tougher route in life. He told me that unfortunately he is the type of person that must learn things the hard way. I was without words when he said that. I have seen many lives begin and end, and everything in between. I was petrified for my son's wellbeing. He was heading down the wrong path and I was worried about him.

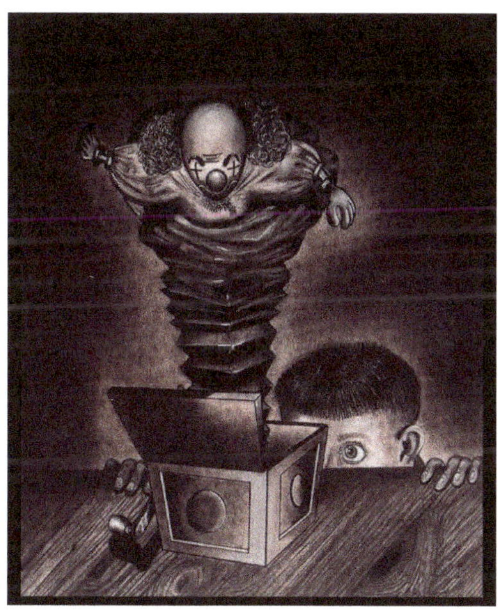

A BOY AND HIS BOX (2001)

This charcoal on paper drawing shows a boy taking chances and discovering new things.

Chapter 15

Orphaned

If things could not get worse, my older brother Liam showed up at my door out of nowhere, unannounced. I used to get him weed, but I hadn't heard from him in a while at that point. When I answered the door, he quickly blurred out "Mom is in the hospital, and she might die". I was instantly confused and then quickly thought he was crazy and I'm sure she's fine. After all I was raised to not totally trust him. But nope, he was indeed correct.

There was a lot of tension between Mom and Liam over the years. They were both difficult people, I think. I felt as though he might have been there to make sure she made it into the dirt. But it is not fair for me to judge their relationship. I believe that their terrible relationship led to a lot of Liam's challenges in life. Once again, I can only speculate.

Liam, like all of us in the family delt with some sort of mental health challenge one way or another. He had always felt like he needed to prove himself. Show that he is good or the best at something. He was in nursing school at the time, and he was displaying some of the skills he had learned. He was challenging the hospital staff's knowledge, and it appeared as though he was showing off a little. At the same time, he seemed to genuinely care. It was upsetting though. My head was not clear, it was a tough time. I just wanted to be left alone to process what was happening.

Even though it had been eight years since my father died, it felt as though I had just gone through it. I was now going through this pain again with my mother. At fifty-nine, she was even younger than my father was when he died. I was at the hospital every day. I taped a picture of my kids, her grandkids to the railing of her hospital bed next to her face. She opened her eyes involuntarily at times. I thought maybe she would still be able to see and catch a glimpse of their faces and it would give her the power to fight, if she had any fight left in her. Liam brought a radio, and I played music for her. I mainly played my parents' song, from when they first met, "My Eyes Adored You". It was their song.

All the tests came back and proved that she was brain dead. Once again, I had the emotional task of making the final decision of removing yet another parent from Life support, or she would wither away in a vegetative state. The most disturbing for me was when the hospital priest came into the room and read her Last-Rites. There were a few family members around the bed, her brothers, and some of her kids.

Right in the middle of the priest praying over her slowly dying body, Liam decided to reach over and suction out her airway. It was so upsetting. Her body jerked and the noises she made are unforgettable. Everyone was in shock, the priest even paused for a second and then kept reading. When everyone left, I said something to him. “Can you just be her son, there are already here people paid to take care of her”. He did not like what I said, he just walked away.

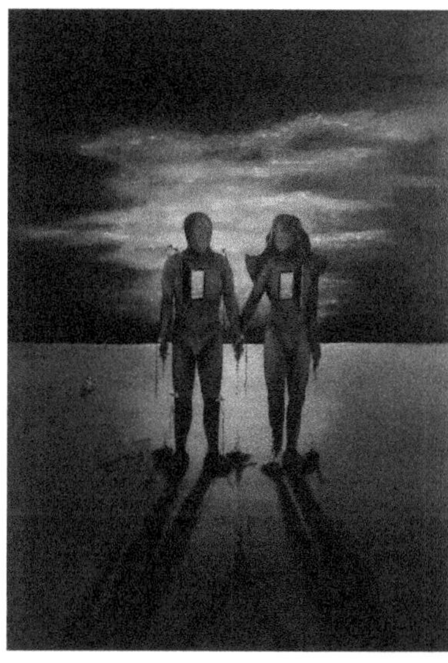

BROKEN HOME
(2012)

This oil on canvas surreal Painting expresses the pain of loss.

Later that night they removed mom’s life support. My mother and I were alone in the hospital room. She was hanging on for a while. I talked to her and held her hand. I dozed off for just a few minutes, and then I felt a tap on my shoulder. It was a nurse. She said bluntly, “She’s dead.”, just like that. She said that my mom was waiting for me to fall to sleep so she could leave. I remember walking to my car and just sitting in it and thinking for a while. I went home that night sad as to be expected. I was glad that I was able to be with her when she left, she wasn’t alone. I called Liam to let him know mom was dead, and he refused to speak to me, and it stayed that way.

I had a tough time accepting that she just dropped dead at fifty-nine without warning. I continued to ask questions. This one nurse took me aside and consoled me. I wish I knew her name. She was the only one that thought I deserved to know something, or maybe she was sick of hearing me ask. She simply asked me a question. She said, "Mom had a tough life, right?". I replied "Yes, she sure did". Then she said, "Life just got to her". Still not knowing exactly what that meant, deep down I understood well. Later looking at medical records I read that she had a bunch of different substances in her system. Although the death certificate stated, "Respiratory Distress."

I was always told that I was planned. On my mother's death bed, Uncle James found it necessary to inform me that my father knocked her up by accident. That he didn't know what to do. In fact, my mother was going to abort me. James put his hand on my father's shoulder and said, "Congratulations, ya going to get married and have a baby," My uncle James was a tough guy. My father was a quiet, peaceful man.

My father did love my mother, but he was probably nervous after being screwed over in that past already. Having a family and having it taken away. She always said that she wanted me. I guess she did because she kept me. I think my father wasn't completely ready for a lifetime commitment yet. He was just dating a pretty, young girl with long brown hair and big boobs. Now he was committed. Even though he was afraid, he also wanted a family deep down. After all it was his life dream. I think he saw the red flags early on and that's what frightened him. It's amazing how life works. The introduction of a sister to a friend. A few decisions later and BAM! Here I am today writing this book half a century later.

I personally never saw excessive drinking, thank God. He called himself a former alcoholic. I don't know if he was using the term loosely or if he truly was an alcoholic. I don't think he drank like that though. I think that maybe he drank every day after work like many to unwind. Maybe too much at times probably… right, or wrong. He was probably called an alcoholic and started to believe he was. Everyone has their crutch, I guess. I wasn't born yet, so I couldn't really say.

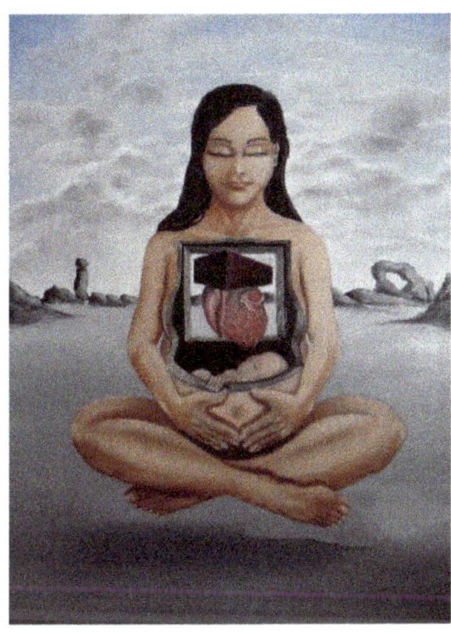

BIRTH
(2012)

This oil on canvas painting was one in a series of Surreal artworks. I was still discovering who I was as an artist., Experimenting and studying the masters.

When I went to my mother's apartment to clean it out. I went through my father's personal belongings when he died, and here I was not that long after, going through my mother's personal things. Except this time, I needed to clean and empty out her apartment completely. I remember walking in and seeing her last few cigarette cigarettes, with the butts in the ashtray. Signs of the last things she ate. On the fridge was a drawing that my daughter drew for her recently before that.

I brought my daughter with me to my mother's apartment. It was her first time there because my mother just moved in not long before that. My daughter was only five years old, and very smart. She looked around this new place for the first time and said, "This is Grandma's house, and where is grandma". I said she had to go somewhere. My daughter replied with, "she died didn't she". It was sad. She lost her last grandmother and would grow up without one just like me.

There were scavengers asking for stuff. They seem to know what they were asking for. This couple had obviously been to my mother's apartment before. They were young. They were probably the ones that were enabling her with what eventually participated in her death. It was whatever at that point. She had nothing to do, her life really sucked. My dad was dead eight years. She really had no family anymore. Everyone abandoned her. I didn't, but I also wasn't there all the time either. So, she wanted to get high. I probably would have done the same. She really did not have a reason not to.

Before my father died, he got them into a nice place. Nicest affordable living apartment I had ever seen. It was like a condominium in the middle of a park. A few years after my father died, she was kicked out for fighting and ended up back in Central Falls where we started thirty-five years prior. She was a mess ever since my father died, getting into trouble. I have bailed her out of jail for shoplifting. She would be bored, walk into a store, fill the carriage up and wheel it right out the door. She did not have a car, so she pushed that carriage all the way home. She was banned from every convenience store in the area.

I carried a lot of guilt. I was there but I could have given her a little more reason to live. I could have made her life a little better by spending more time with her. I was not capable emotionally. I did the best I could at that time. I was there for her. I was present for her, helping her especially when my dad first died. I did not abandon her. I just think that I could have done better.

One more Uncle James sighting when mom died. He came up from Vegas to do I'm not sure what. He left before she even took her last breath. He didn't go to my mother's funeral. He said, "I don't do funerals". I wonder why. He didn't like seeing dead people, I guess. I felt bad to be honest because she really thought the world of him. In the end, he wasn't there for her. They were once very close. Growing up, she always talked about him. She worshipped him because he was the one who taught her survival skills. He taught her the streets.

I had to scramble and figure out how I was going to manage her burial. Nothing was planned and she had no life insurance. Liam was the oldest of us four. He said he would help me, but I never saw or heard from him again after that night at the hospital. I made sure she had a proper sendoff anyway. Katrina was more helpful with this death than my father's. I think it was because she personally experienced the death of her father a couple years prior. She probably

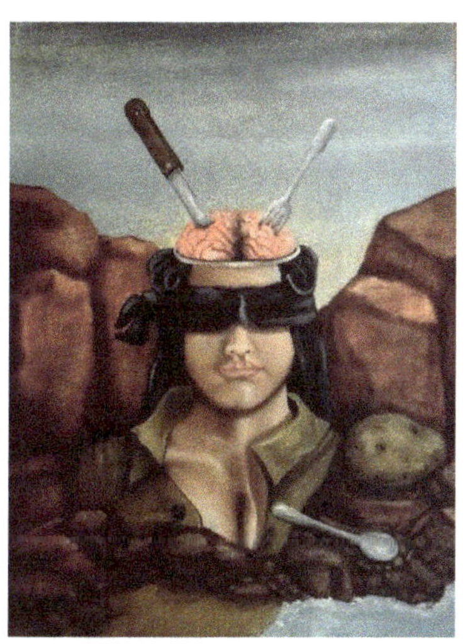

WATCHING SUFFER
(2012)

This oil on canvas painting expresses my mother's struggle with her mental health.

understood better how painful it is.

Several people at the pre-funeral showing said my mother looked so pretty and looked great. It was nice of them to try, and be kind, but it was kind of annoying. I was thinking, "She's dead and she looks terrible." But I get it, death is a difficult thing to process, even for the guest paying respect. I was still in shock because that was the second parent to drop dead without warning.

The day of the funeral my sister told me that I was a good son to our mother. That meant a lot to me, more than she probably realized. Besides myself, she was the only sibling to show up for the funeral. My friends Josh and Jimmy were there to help carry my mother's casket. Helping me carry my mother to the hole in the ground in which she was to be buried. In life they were both my closest friends.

Seeing both my parents' caskets carried directly to the hole in the ground that they lay in is another image that burnt into my mind. The cemetery tries to make it clean. They draped artificial grass over the sidewalls of the hole, and the pile of dirt next to it. I was trying to process my mother's unexpected death. Both of my parents were dead. It was a very lonely feeling. I didn't realize how empty it would feel with my parents gone. I was dealing with it all alone, emotionally and financially.

I was trying to process the mixed feelings of anger and mourning. My father was sixty-seven when he died. I was only twenty-nine. Eight years later my mother died at only fifty-nine. Both seemed to be healthy and full of energy. Suddenly they both dropped dead, and both were brought back to life. I watched over them both for days in the hope they would break out of what appeared to be a coma. Watching their eyes open and close. I still believed each time I saw their eyes open that they might be waking up that time, but they never did. leaving me with the responsibility of removing their life support. This destroyed me, how bad I was still yet to realize.

I was their only child together. I grew up with them. A big part of me was suddenly gone. My daughter had her grandma for just five years. My mother would become a foggy memory that my stories and a few photos keep alive. My dad never met her, she was born after he passed. They both left me the same way unexpectedly; I was traumatized ten times over. I was a broken person.

It really sucks when a parent dies young. Only as wiser adults do we really start to truly understand life. We grow up and realize that our parents are just people too. Realizing that we all mess up from time to time. I envy people my age and older that still have their parents. I think old people are the most interesting of humans. Think about your own experiences, ups and downs in life so far. Imagine that plus another 20-50 years of more life-changing experiences. Old people have seen some shit in life. They deserve the upmost respect, especially from the younger people.

I wish my parents were still alive. I would love to have an adult conversation with them. I'd tell them that I understand. They were just people trying to survive with the foundation they were given to build on. It's a vicious cycle that takes strength to break. It's been my mission to be that person.

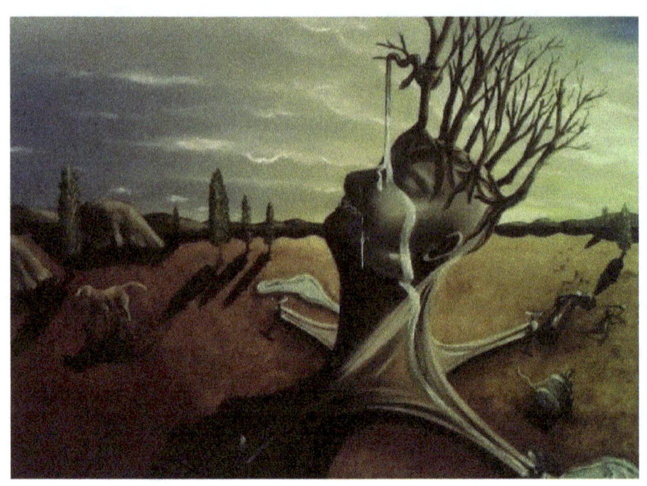

TEARS
(2012)
A visual of racing thoughts, confusion and fear.

" Life does not come with an instruction manual. We spend the first half of our life writing one, and we spend the second half of our life trying to follow it".

-Me

Chapter 16

Moving Forward

I started studying art more, the masters, and their styles. I took an interest in their background after taking a few art history classes at the local state college. I took an interest in Salvador Dali. It has been said that one must study the masters, to be a true artist. I created a series of Surreal oil paintings inspired by Dali's style. I appreciated the abstract creativity while he still captured realism with his smooth brush strokes. Those paintings were heavily inspired by my childhood and the emotional pain I was feeling at the time.

The charcoal drawings and surreal oil paintings are what brought me to my first gallery showing. It felt amazing yet scary to have my art on the walls of a gallery. I felt as though I was progressing. That seemed to be what the artist aims for, gallery showings. The scary part is putting yourself out there like that. People are judging you and your talent. I've seen a lot of people and even a few famous people stand in front of my artwork for a couple minutes to absorb it. It feels really good to see people appreciate your talent.

Shortly after, I booked more shows and then had my first

show in New York. I didn't have a lot of paintings, but I had enough to show, and people liked them. It was inspiring and motivating. I came a long way from years ago when I showed my artwork for the first time to the lady at the gallery in providence. I did not plan to keep creating surreal paintings. At the time I was still testing my own self. I always appreciated artwork that wasn't simple and obvious. I enjoy work that stimulates the mind and makes one think.

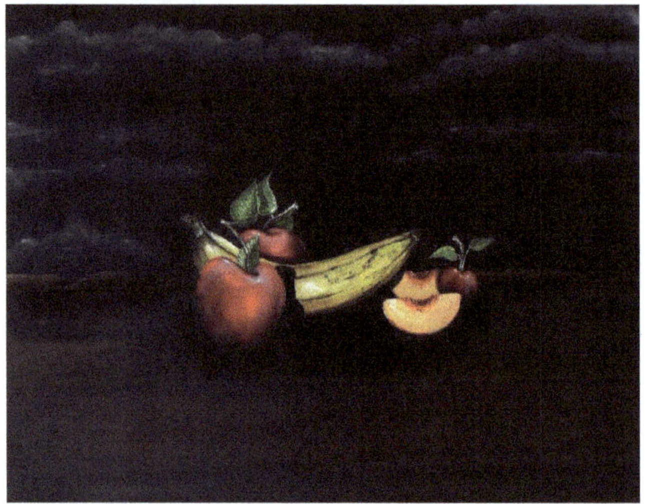

FRUIT
(2012)

This oil painting leans towards realism, yet surrealism due to not being what it first appears to be. A test of techniques and skill level at that time.

As an artist, I was still discovering myself. I was also proving things to myself. So, I have done some realism, portraits, still life and landscapes. But I don't enjoy it as much. It's abstract work that I enjoy creating. The freedom! We had cameras to Capture what already exist. I wanted to invent new things. It was part of my process. I was still learning art, and even bigger I was still learning who I was as a person and who I was as an artist.

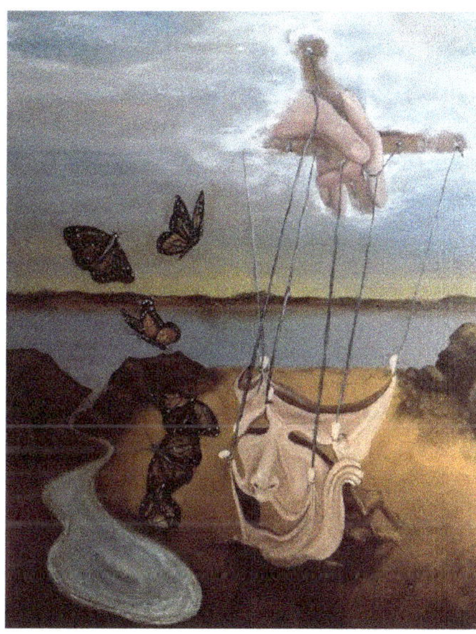

MEDICATION
(2012)

This surreal oil on canvas painting displays the tides that always go up and down, hiding behind a mask.

Living as close to a normal life as possible, or at least in my mind. I was committed to not allowing myself to crumble. Besides art, I was living life... Putting my best foot forward. I had a routine being a dad. I was also a growing artist but had a regular job still, that I went to five days a week to make a living and provide.

It was one cold winter morning heading into work when I pulled into the parking lot at work, preparing for a day of work. I stepped out of my truck and without warning, my feet instantly flew up in the air and I landed on my back. The parking lot was not salted, and it was covered in black ice. I hurt myself. I was out of work, and in pain. I had some extra time on my hands. I was thinking about my life, and I started creating a lot. The pain meds made that possible. I'd get a few hours of relief and that allowed me to paint.

If it wasn't for my youngest daughter who was little at the time, I don't know what direction I would have taken. She kept me thinking as clearly as I could. She was the one thing that I was not going to mess up with. I was determined to be the best dad I could. There was always a feeling as though she needed me more than an average kid needs their dad, and I was not going to let her down. I was judged and ridiculed for being too nice to her.

I took her to the playground just about every nice day after work. Sometimes to two, if the first was overcrowded. We did a bunch of stuff together. We had the best times. Driving Go Karts and going to Mystic aquarium was always a fun daddy daughter day in the summer. I remember once I took her to a petting zoo, and there were signs up that said, "Don't pet the animals." We got a good laugh out of that one. We always made it home for the ice cream man. Hanging out with my daughter was my favorite thing to do.

I continued to paint even more. I started with acrylics, and then went to oils. I had a lot of time on my hands being out of work with my back issues from the fall at work. Time for my daughter and time to paint. I had a tough time sleeping and was painting my ass off until the late hours of the night, early hours of the morning when my daughter was sleeping.
I was embracing the skills I learned along the way. I attended art school as an adult. Utilizing what I learned as a kid at those Rhode Island School of Design workshops. Growing up I watched my dad sketch, and my mom showed me color. I

studied my favorite masters; I paid attention to the artists around me. I knew one thing for sure at this point, art was about being unique.

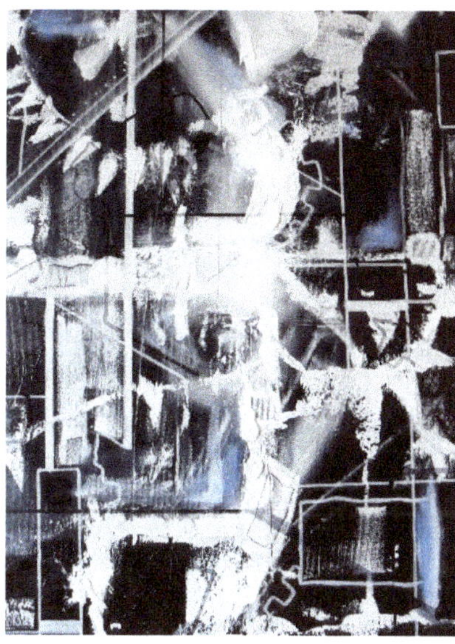

STRUCTURE
(2013)

This acrylic on canvas painting was an aggressive abstract study. Learning to aesthetically arrange shapes to create depth.

There people who create art, and there is an Artist! I knew that I was an Artist because of the way I thought, the way I felt. The way I looked at things, and the reason I created the artworks I had created. I was trying to invent who I was as an artist. Trying to find myself and trying to find my style. A great legacy is what every artist works towards. A legacy is what every man dreams for. I wanted my kids to be proud of me. When I die one day, I need the death notice to list my career as being an artist.

Pain often enhances my creativity; I sure had a lot of creative juices flowing then. Like most artists I started off drawing as a kid. Airbrushing showed me the way and encouraged me to explore different mediums and tools. I studied the master's and grew an appreciation for Surrealism because it challenged my skills and my mind, helping me learn techniques. It was still too confining. I liked the feeling of free thinking. I enjoyed painting aggressively, even incorporating scrapers and anything I saw that I felt could help me create what I imagined. My work became more abstract, but I liked to keep some subject matter present more than often. With that my work changed drastically over time.

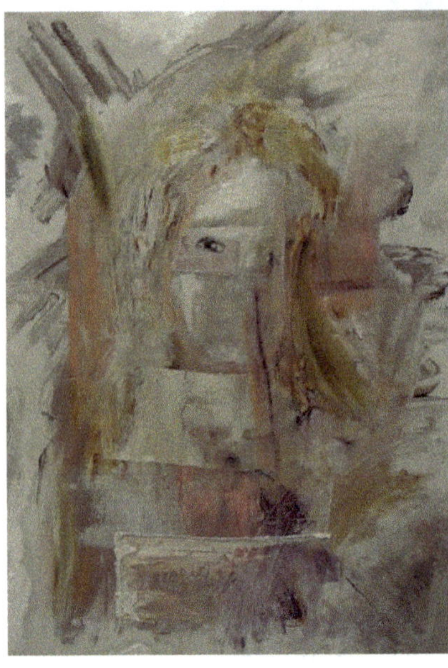

IMAGE OF A GIRL (2013)

This is an aggressively abstracted acrylic on canvas painting incorporating subject matter. The subject in this painting is my youngest daughter.

For me the most satisfying part of being an artist is creating, and that sense of accomplishment. Selling a piece of artwork was never about the money for me. Even though we need it to survive. Knowing that regardless of how much or little the client spent. A person enjoyed the piece I made so much that they want to hang it up and look at it every day and are willing to use their hard-earned money to pay for it. That is a blessing!

A few years back when I was going through my father's things after he died, I found a puzzle of the last supper by

Leonardo DaVinci. It was my dad's when he was younger, it was older than me. It had become a family heirloom. My father and I built it a few times over the years growing up. I decided to build it once again, this time unfortunately without my father. It was a big puzzle, so it took time to build. I was moving some things around and accidentally left it alone unattended with my dog Coco nearby. She got into the unfinished puzzle that I cherished so much, and she destroyed it. It was upsetting and disappointing.

Like any artist I was looking for that invention, something unique. I stumbled across something without really trying. Pieces of the puzzle were everywhere including outside in the yard. I gathered thew pieces and built it and as I feared there were pieces missing. I was heartbroken over it.

That night while painting I took a break. I sat down and stared at the incomplete box of puzzle pieces sitting next to my paint. Still upset over the ruined puzzle that was my dad's. I spontaneously scooped up a handful of puzzle pieces and mixed them with paint. Then I smeared them across a canvas. I did a lot of painting, but this is when I created my very first puzzle composition. People loved it, and I continued to make more. I was determined to be successful.

Some were made with paint, some without, coming up with new ideas as I went along. I obtained a surplus of puzzles, looking for color schemes and images. Separating the colors needed to achieve the looks I was aiming for. Adhering each puzzle piece strategically to the canvas based on color, size, and shape. Mixing multiple puzzles into each one. I started creating compositions that the puzzle pieces were never meant to create.

The puzzle composition was what brought me to my first solo show in Boston. This was the first time I showed my puzzle works, and they were selling. I was doing well. My work appeared in a few magazines and publications. This was the first time an Art Critic came to my basement studio and critiqued my work. She had nothing bad to say, and that was encouraging. The review was positive. She called my puzzle creation a Happy Accident. Until then my parents were the only people to ever be supportive of my art, yet they didn't live long enough to ever see me develop into a real Artist.

HAPPY ACCIDENT (2013)

This is the very first Puzzle composition that was created using acrylic paint and material from my father's puzzle of The Last Supper.

Art has always been a positive escape for me, and the thing I loved most for myself. Art was never Something I did; It was and still is what I am. There is nothing more satisfying to me than the accomplishment of a completed piece of art that I am happy with. It makes me feel good about myself.

I was getting attention for my work. I was progressing and finding who I was as an artist. I was working at it day and night. Most don't realize the logistical and business part of being an artist. It's not all fun in the studio. I was learning that part of it too. It's not easy to get successful artists to show you the way. Being a successful artist is more than often something you need to learn on your own, but I was lucky to find a few good souls along the way to help guide me.

I had given life my best and tried to enjoy the good times when the good times were present. This is just what life was. Art was something that never let me down. I continued to paint and draw but I had something unique happening and I was hopeful, reaching for the stars.

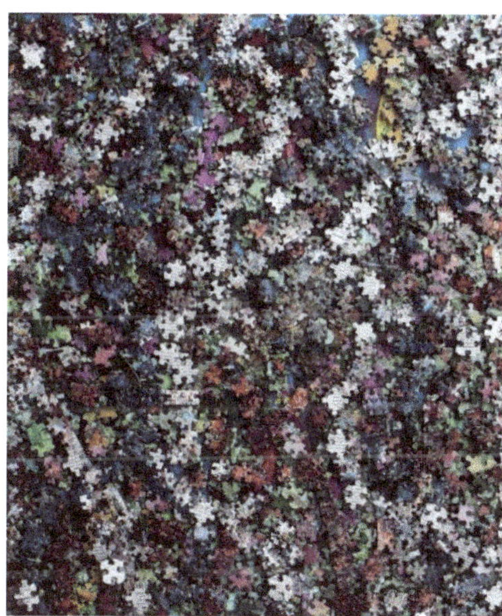

FLOWERGARDEN FROM THE SKY (2013)

Puzzle material on canvas. Discovering many possibilities. Working with colors

Chapter 17

Crossroads, My 40s

There was still a void, something was missing. I never witnessed a normal healthy relationship or had one myself. I lived a life of tolerance and settling. I had been learning how to live a normal life since the day I decided to run away from home at seventeen. I thought I should be happy that someone wanted to be with me. My self-esteem and confidence were challenged. Art was the only thing that helped me feel good about myself.

I watched my father struggle with my mom as she repeatedly told me growing up to never trust a female. So, at this point she was right. I had not met one yet that I could. Even Katrina was loyal and trustworthy in one way, but that is not the only part of a relationship. I couldn't trust her to care about me, a person.

As I became older and wiser, I started to question my life choices, and what role I played in Katrina's life. The things she said caused me to question her sincerity. I felt more like a security blanket because she did not like change. She would rather suffer in silence than take a risk and face the unknown. She was not a nurturer, and I was not loved the way I needed to be loved. So much had happened, and our bond was broken.

Katrina always wanted more things from life, nicer home, nicer car, better vacations. I do not think that she ever saw her lack of contribution towards those goals. I was working a job that I hated in retail management. It was not who I was, but I did what needed to be done. She was blind to the fact that she was never willing to put in the same effort and sacrifice. She simply pointed her finger at me and complained. She seemed to be a miserable person with me; she was obviously unhappy. I see now that she had her own issues that she probably didn't even realize. I wear my feelings on my sleeve, so my emotions are hard to hide. I was emotional and sensitive. She felt putting effort into being nice was not being real, so she refused to be that person. She said, "I'm a realist."

I've had death wished upon me countless times in graphic details. She said things like, "I hope you get into a brutal car accident on the way home that Mangels your body and you die slow." Intimacy became rare; weeks turned into months that would go by at times. I was made to feel dirty if I talked about it and voiced my concerns. That is usually the first thing to go when a relationship is broken. It's important, it's about bonding with someone, the comfort and trusting the other with your most inner self.

The mean things said, the rejection, and the feeling like something was wrong with me was overwhelming. I was told that she never loved me and should never have been together because she cut herself short with me and deserved better. I was judged not on my character. I was measured against others who were more successful than me. Often It made me feel like I was lucky to have her because no one else would want me.

We didn't spend quality time together. Katrina slept a lot and slept on the couch every night as she had been doing for a long time. She often seemed angry, and extremely unhappy. It ultimately caused me to be less happy myself as time went on. She would tell me to my face how this guy did this, and this girl's husband got her that, and she spent her time wishing that I were things I was not. She hurt my feelings a lot. In my opinion she was one of those glass half empty kind of people. I became bitter and confused about my mixed feelings. I had my daughter and my art to get me by. Those two things weighed heavily in my life.

I was dealing with severe pain, but it allowed me extra time with my daughter, which was great. She was having challenges with her emotions, anxiety, and depression. Me being able to spend more time with her was going to be beneficial to her emotional development. The accident was a blessing in disguise. Although the pain left me with limitations for a little while.

I was able to spend a significant amount of time with my daughter that most dads do not get. She was not getting along well with her mother and her mother was not always managing her behavior well either. It was becoming a vicious cycle. She would appear to have patience at first but let it build up until she burst like a tea kettle. There was a lot of screaming and a huge lack of a filter. Katrina was vicious with her mouth. Way more painful than any swings at me could ever be. It seemed as though she could not help herself.

After years of living in an angry environment, I became somewhat of an angry person myself. I struggled to be the seemingly happy person that my daughter needed me to be. I remember being so depressed and her walking over to me saying, "Daddy," and I turned around towards her and would automatically put on a fake smile as I responded to her. Seeing her adorable little face did make it a little easier to smile when I looked at her. She was the apple of my eye. I took being her daddy seriously.

She was the first child that I was given the opportunity to completely raise from beginning to end. I love my older daughter Tammy and son Jr, but I was unfortunately pushed away early on. I was a great father to them, especially until Rhonda and I got divorced a while back. I was younger when they were born and earned less money. I was a good provider and loving father to them as well though.

When your child grows up in a different home and you don't have a decent relationship with the mother, it becomes extremely difficult for the parent to live separately. No matter what, you never seem to be doing enough in other's eyes. The parent with the child does not understand that feeling, or the challenge the other has. The child only knows what they hear being said, and they are primarily hearing what the parent they live with is saying mostly, while their judgment is jaded.

I had Tammy and Jr. every weekend, I paid child support and still bought some things like coats, clothes, and shoes when I could. We went to the movies, amusement parks, beaches, etc. But I wasn't able to tuck them into bed at night, or sit at the table for dinner, or help with homework. That creates a void. Tammy suffered the most because she was only two years old and does not remember me ever living with her. If she only realized how much I loved her, and still do!

She was quiet and distant. I did not know how to handle that. I just went with the flow. I know she heard a lot; her mother and I were not on the best terms. I was afraid to put pressure on her and scare her away even more. She had a little sister now. But having a new baby also meant that I was sharing my free time with a third child that was much younger. I did my best. Sometimes your best still isn't good enough.

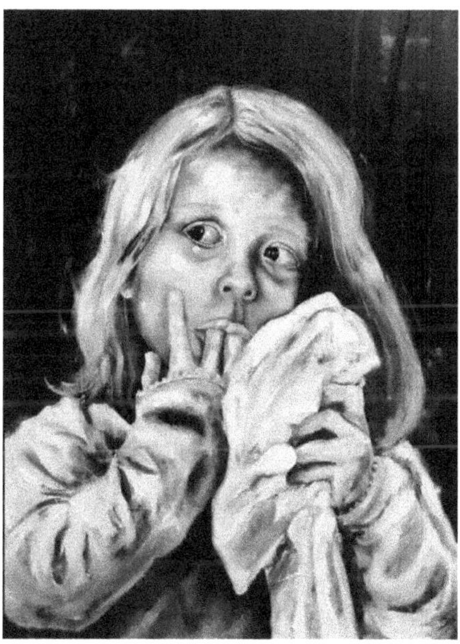

INNOCENCE

(2012)

This acrylic on canvas painting of my youngest daughter was finger painted.

The physical pain from the accidents was unbearable, and I was prescribed morphine pills and that's where I allowed myself to slip a little. I was incredibly unhappy with life in general, filled with guilt. A lot had happened, and I was losing the ability to cope. The marriage was beyond challenged. To top it off I was in a lot of pain. Then for whatever reason my doctor told me not to chew the morphine pills, not that I was even going to think of doing that.

I wasn't attracted to drugs or getting high like that. One rough day I did what I was told not to do. I wanted them to hit faster, not realizing that I chewed time release pills. It didn't seem to make me feel high, but something made me do it again for some reason. It helped my mood and with my creativity that first time. Once everyone was in bed sleeping, I painted all night long. It was getting a hold of me, and I didn't even see it happening. It was like a silent high. I didn't really feel it, I just felt better.

I did not do drugs. I had hard drugs like heroin shoved in my face countless times for free, and I never touched them. I didn't even see it coming. I had other pain meds for my injuries and did not abuse them at all. I had less tolerance for bullshit. Katrina's attitude towards me often made me feel like I was not good enough. Talking about how great other women's husbands were, the better jobs they had and the places they went. She often threw in my face that I was like my crazy mother, who was dead at that point.

The truth is that she destroyed what I felt for her. After all those years she still didn't know me. She never took the time to listen with empathy. If she knew me, she would have appreciated me for who I was. Maybe she would have been even more disappointed with the notion that I was as good as I was going to get. She was not truly happy with who I was, and her actions turned me against her in the process. Until I sold my first painting Katrina consistently threw in my face how I've wasted money on art supplies yet never sold a painting. It was hurtful. She claimed to be supportive because she allowed me to buy art supplies. In fact, she felt it was a waste of money and I was chasing a fantasy. She made sure I knew that every time she was angry with me. She never understood that I was learning my craft, and an artist was who I was.

I struggled with depression, anxiety and flashbacks of traumatic situations from my past, but my daughter's little face made me smile, and creating art was therapeutic. I always enjoyed going for a ride listening to the music as loud as possible. Twelve-inch subwoofers banging in the trunk. Feeling the music was and still is therapeutic for me. The type of music I listen to depends on what I am doing. I have always been sensitive to music. Some songs make me drive faster, and some slow me down. Music with a slow tempo can trigger tears. I like energetic music of any kind. Eminem was an artist I could always relate to. WU-Tang Clan were artists that I also enjoyed painting too. They got my creativity racing, and just filled me with energy, and still do.

I was creating a lot of art at that time, still exploring new styles. Art was my escape. I was painting, but very focused on developing the puzzle compositions. Creating out of emotion as I usually did. I was not interested in making pretty pictures. Katrina always told me to paint landscapes and water scenes because that's what sold. She did not understand that I was an Artist in every sense of the word. I was expressing myself on canvas, documenting my feelings. I think she just didn't get that.

I decided to look for an art agent and came across this guy named Donny. He ended up not being an agent, but he became a friend and a mentor. He had experience. He had sold high dollar art in auctions. He reassured me that I had talent and encouraged me. Even though I had already started painting, he inspired me to pursue being a Fine Artist. I painted with him a few times. I did a lot of listening. He taught me a lot in a short time, and he attended my shows.

Donny gave me a case of canvases once and asked me to paint him one painting as a thank you. I gave him back a black and white portrait of himself that I finger painted. He helped me Network, introducing me to new people in the art world. He had many ups and downs in his own personal life, so we could relate well. I will always stay in touch with him. He was the first established artist that ever gave me the right time of day.

I've dabbled in different mediums over the years. I started learning basic techniques as a child attending Rhode Island School of Design, I did graffiti and airbrushing in my teens through my thirties. I also accepted commissions from companies as large as ESPN. I airbrushed a lot. A radio DJ gave me the opportunity to collaborate with him on a project as he interviewed various music artists. I created a bunch of stuff for celebrities. One celebrity that I personally worked with was a music artist from The Wu Tang Clan. He came to perform in Providence one time, and I was invited to go up onstage with him. It was a fun experience, we became friendly. It was a night I'll never forget.

I gained interest in writing, and I wrote for and illustrated a kid's page in a local newspaper for a while. The smaller projects all taught me lessons that made me who I am today as an artist. I was progressively growing as a fine artist from my thirties through my forties. I started a graphic T-shirt business but never had the funding for marketing. I even started tattooing at one point, and instantly was not bad at it, but I didn't love it either. Still searching for a medium I could make money with. I had a good job at the cell phone store but kept working towards the goal of being a fulltime artist only. I continuously searched for something to do in art that would earn enough to pay the bills, although Fine Art is what my passion was.

Things were looking good. I was in a few publications, paper magazine and digital, getting all good reviews. Gallery shows from New York through Rhode Island were booked. My work was shown virtually overseas in London. I did a bunch of small projects. I was finally selling fine art and people were starting to know who I was. I had paintings hanging in homes and offices all over the country. I was starting to make a name for myself, gaining recognition. I was obsessed with art and my hard work was starting to pay off.

Even with these successes, I was still very unhappy with my personal life. I was lonely. I was hurt because I felt rejected and like less of a person at home. I was not doing ok at all. I began tattooing myself. At one point the pain from the tattoo machine became an escape from the emotional pain I was feeling inside.

I was practically living in my basement studio painting myself to death. I would get a few hours' sleep and then wake up to take care of my daughter. I spent the day with her, and then I went back to painting again at night when she was sleeping. That was pretty much what I was doing every day. There was a point when I guess one could say things caught up with me. I felt myself deteriorating mentally. Someone new moved in across the street. She was friendly, she had a daughter too, who played together with mine. So, talking wasn't so unusual. Then quickly she became very friendly. She admired my artwork. It innocently made me feel good about myself. I felt neglected at home for many years and led to believe that

I was less than others for so long. The attention was refreshing. She eventually told me that she fell for me. I didn't feel the same, but I loved the lift in self-confidence.

I'm ashamed of it, my inability to think clearly at that time. Somewhere along the way I teleported mentally into a shit show. I was a mess emotionally, and she saw that. She was very pushy. She knew I was unhappy and was mentally unstable. We didn't sleep together, but she was working on it. The girl started to like me too much too fast, and that was scary. Quickly realizing that it was a mistake even allowing myself to feel better around her. My built-up bitterness with Katrina got us to that point.

I'm not a sneaky person, so I wasn't good at hiding things. Even though we weren't intimate, I knew the friendship with her was still not ok. It did not last more than a couple of weeks before Katrina came across messages that I was getting. She called me and told me to get my things and leave. I tried to talk to her, but she didn't want to hear it. Nothing had actually happened. I was not trying to leave Katrina; my daughter was still way too young. This was not supposed to happen. I didn't want it to.

My parents were dead, I had no place to go. I had no money for a hotel. I started acting without thinking, and things were getting out of control. This was not planned, and it was unraveling poorly. I wasn't in love; this was not the person for me either, I wasn't trying to be with her, cheat, or do anything. I was absorbing positive energy from someone that made me feel better about myself. That was my mistake, then I was stuck with nowhere to go, so I stayed at the girl's house for a few days, and I realized when it was too late that it was totally inappropriate. I should have slept in my car. I was broken and had no idea how to process what was happening or how to handle it properly.

Katrina had been telling me for a long time that I was mentally ill like my mother, and I needed help. With all my wild ideas of being an artist, associating with rappers, acting "to young", as she said. Then there was my depression and anxiety, to a degree she was right. I was definitely struggling mentally. I think she was misinterpreting the situation and what led to it though. I was so confused, and my head started spinning.

I was totally overwhelmed, and eventually admitted myself into the hospital. My first night was in detox. Come to find out I luckily didn't get to the point of having an addiction to the Morphine pills, I nipped it in the bud just in time. Although, they were enough to take my already screwed up head and through me through a loop. Temporarily destroying my life.

I was told that one night I was walking in the middle of the street at two in the morning and no one could get me in the car. I don't remember any of that. I was told that I was in an ambulance, that I also don't remember. When I was removed from detox, I was put into a mental health unit. The same one that I learned to play pool with many years prior when I was visiting my mother there when I was a kid. I was in the hospital for twenty-two days in all. I do clearly remember that part though.

Katrina excessively expressed my family's mental health history to the doctors. Especially my late mother's bipolar, and any actions I made that she felt were bipolar like symptoms. It made sense to the doctor, since my family history with it is strong. The doctor came back with a diagnosis of bipolar. Not saying she was wrong, but it was heavily suggested. Katrina convinced me and the doctor that I needed more meds to be stable. Doses were increased. To be honest, the most important thing was that I remained in my daughter's life fulltime until she was grown. I was sacrificing everything to make sure she had me in her life. I knew that Katrina would turn her against me if I was not.

Katrina read a lot about psych meds so when she talked to the doctors, she seemed to know her shit, and she did to a point. But with what intentions is the question. Whose agenda? In my opinion she was pulling strings on what medicines they were giving me, and taking away what she didn't want me to have. At one point I was a zombie doing what I was told, full of guilt, looking for forgiveness. I agree that I definitely had issues, but some of what she saw as a mental health problem was just me being me. The fact is, she didn't like everything about me from the start.

I have lots of memories from being locked in the hospital. One person that I never forgot about from the that place was Julie. She had autism and severe depression. She was so nice and in so much pain. One night I saw her crying. I sat down with her and asked her what was wrong. I listen to her talk as I drew her a picture. Many years later she contacted me on social media and told me that I saved her life from suicide that night. She had planned on killing herself until I sat with her as I drew her a picture.

The experience itself was therapeutic. I met a lot of nice, damaged people and that was the biggest therapy of all, and it was humbling. My head was becoming clearer, and I felt bad about myself. Not feeling bad for myself, but about myself. I resented my mother for so much and I realized then that she was only human. Thankfully I didn't subject my kids to nearly as much as my mother did.

I left the hospital heavily medicated. Even though I was doing well with my art before this all happened, the goal of being an accomplished artist became nothing more than a figment of my imagination. Caused by my mental illness and mania. Things were said that led to believe I had crazy unrealistic ideas and was just unstable. Normal people didn't have these aspirations and create art all the time. I stopped painting, airbrushing, tattooing, and every form of art I was doing. In fact, I sold all my equipment and supplies, everything. For the first time in my life, I gave up on art. Just as I was starting to get somewhere.

Katrina said she understood her mistakes, and I recognized my own. She promised to put effort into the relationship. Her efforts wore off quickly though. Even though I wasn't planning to leave her, the separation happened. This was the second time we separated, and she went back on her promises. At this point in her life, she should have known that she wasn't capable. We were too different, and she would never be happy with me, and she would intern make me unhappy as well. Which in return made me even more incapable of making her happy. It was a vicious cycle.

The only positive thing that came from this was that for some reason she became less violent. Physical incidents became rarer, which was nice. I think she was afraid I would leave again. This helped make life more tolerable at home. She did not want to be forced into changes. I feel that it was more comfortable for her to tolerate and settle for me, who I believe she didn't really like. I was medicated and numb,

Staring at walls with no feelings. I concluded that I had to make myself happy and the key was not a better relationship. It was about being able to tolerate the relationship. I was finding ways to make myself happy.

I felt so low. I felt like scum, I hated myself at that point. I became a mentally ill man that should be grateful that my mistakes were forgiven… sort of. As I was told all the time over and over by her. Things got a little crazy for a while. There was a lot of moving around. We ended up letting the house go that Katrina grew up in. It was a joint decision. We raised my daughter there and I had a lot of good memories with big birthdays thrown for her. Swing sets, pools and bouncy castles. The house that was purchased from Katrina's mom was falling apart faster than I could fix it. The neighborhood was falling apart even faster and was infested with rats that were getting in.

I found this cute little house for us not far away and in a nice neighborhood. The lady did not want to rent it to us at first. There were a few factors. For one I was not working and was getting long-term disability from the company I had worked for. We went back and forth for days. Finally, I told her, "Listen I'll give you first month, security and last month". This was a lot of money and then I told her, from that point on I would pay rent a month earlier every month going forward. Always paying a month in advance. So, she went for it, she let us move in. It was a relief.

The kicker was… No pets allowed. The property owner didn't allow dogs. Coco was fifteen years old, she was full of lumps, had difficulties eating and she was showing signs of pain. We had to make a difficult decision. We had let the house we owned go. It was being foreclosed on and we needed to move out.

When we first got our dog Coco, she was a puppy that was taken from her mom too soon. I came home from work one day and there she was. I never had a dog before, so that was a learning experience. She was a cute pit, lab mix. She had serious behavioral issues. She was mean to everyone but the three people including myself living within the four walls of the house. Even jumped through the glass window to attack the mailman once. She was a couple years old when my youngest daughter was born. When she first came home, I thought I might have needed to get rid of the dog. I had to keep her in the bathroom, and she was tied up a lot unfortunately for a while.

Eventually she calmed down and ended up being great with the baby. I tried hard to not let her go because I knew her chances of finding a nice steady home were going to be slim and she would have probably been put to sleep as a puppy. I actually liked the dog and didn't want anything bad to happen to her.

Then there we were fifteen years later, facing the agonizing decision of letting Coco live a little longer sickly or get my child into a nice stable home from which we could build. I am a parent first! Bringing Coco to the Vet was heartbreaking. I held her as she took her last breath. She just became limp quickly and it was over. Walking in with her and walking out without her. Participating in the last breath of loved ones had become an unfortunate trend in my life.

I was trying to make good for everything, providing a nice home. I had us in a nicer house than ever before. I thought things might work out after all. I was trying to make good for things that had happened. Like things weren't challenging enough I got a letter in the mail telling me that my disability check was ending. They felt as though I could work due to photos taken of me. In the pictures I seemed to be walking normally without pain. They were not considering the medication I was taking for the pain that gave me short periods of relief. Plus, some days are better than others.

I had no income anymore, and I just promised this lady that I would pay the rent early every month. I just begged this lady to trust me. We lived in the house for only one month. To top it off, it was Christmas time. I had just put up a tree and I had no money to put gifts under it or afford the roof over it. The depression was setting in. I don't know what was worse, the sadness or the fear. After all, I just recently left the Psychiatric hospital a few months prior. I wasn't doing so good, but I hid it well.

The landlady was so understanding. She never gave me a hard time when I told her what had happened. She even gave me back my security deposit after only one month. She knew I needed it in the worse way. She felt bad and told me if I ever needed a house and was doing well that I could come back. She did not have to do that at all. The one-year lease I broke off in one month was reason enough to keep my security deposit. She unfortunately got screwed but she knew sincerely it was not my fault. Luckily, the house we owned was still our property... temporarily. We had to move back into it again.

I felt so bad and as though I was a crazy person that destroyed everything. I could not find a job and we had a limited amount of time in this house before the bank was going to auction it off. We couldn't stay. We were facing homelessness. I had never been so scared in my life. I had a bad back, and I was covered in tattoos which were a lot less acceptable at the time.

It was Christmas time. I was overqualified for most jobs available. It was not an excuse to not find a job because God knows I tried and tried hard. I woke up early and started hunting every single day. I searched for work online and on foot. I started praying more and praying hard. Begging God for forgiveness and begging for the ability to fix this disaster I caused for my own selfish reasons. I was looking to be satisfied with life, in fact I made life unbearable for everyone.

I was Chain smoking one cigarette after another because I quit smoking weed. A lot of jobs drug tested, and weed was considered one of those disqualifying drugs then, it was still illegal. I also stopped taking my meds because I was afraid of false negatives when drug screening for jobs. That was probably not a good idea in retrospect. But I could not risk losing out on the opportunity to be hired. I also couldn't tell the employer that I was taking things like Lithium. The tattoos were enough of a problem as it was.

It was a traumatizing experience. Not because I was worried about my own wellbeing. I had others that I just dragged down with me. My main concern was my little girl, she was still a kid and dependent on me to take care of her. Failing her was always a fear.

I recall walking down Thayer Street in Providence. It was raining and I was wearing shoes that were two sizes too big for me, trying to find a job doing anything. After a short time, I was so desperate and so scared that I would have been thrilled to find a job washing dishes. I was wearing make-up and bandages every day to cover my tattoos, trying to disguise my history and hide the evidence of my past. It was one of the most discouraging times in my life.

I did what I always do, I started making plans. How was I going to handle the worst-case scenario, homelessness. For years we lived in a crappy house, but it was ours. My daughter did not know the difference. All she knew was she had her own house with a big back yard, swing set, pool, and a dog. It was all gone. Even the dog was gone. I felt so awful.

I made a list of things I would need to survive in my truck. Items like wet wipes, a bucket, water, foods I could eat on the go. I would go to the gym to shower. This would have made it even harder to get on my feet with no home. if the truck broke down, I'd be in big trouble. Katrina was going to stay at her cousin's house with my daughter... maybe. Jr and Tammy said that they couldn't help me, but they would make sure that their little sister would be safe. I was grateful for that at least. I had not created any art in a while, so I had no outlet. It was one struggle after another.

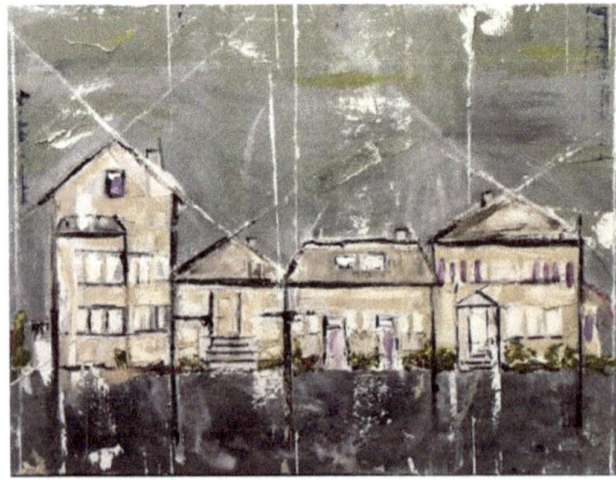

HOMES

(2017)

This oil on canvas abstracted expressionism displays the different places I've called home in past years.

I once believed that I would make it, and even do well one day. I had faith in that idea. We are taught from day one that hard work pays off and we can be anything we wanted to be. I had the mindset that those ideas were for me too. I just had a rough start and little foundation to start building on. It was going to be harder for me and take a little more effort to make this all happen. I was focused with a sense of urgency, yet I was still failing terribly. Almost like there was a force working against me.

Being a failure that caused damage beyond repair is an awful feeling. It gets scary when you start to believe that you are the pain, and your loved ones are better off without you. When your brain is not clear. When suicide becomes a selfless act in your own head, rather than the selfish act it actually is. It got to a point where I thought everyone was better off without me. I had been struggling my entire life, and I was at the end of my rope. It just went too far.

I truly hated myself, I couldn't live with myself anymore. My faith was being challenged. I was going through withdrawals from my psychiatric meds that I went off without weaning. I had insomnia and the most crippling anxiety and depression ever. It had gotten to the point where I had planned my suicide in detail. I kept a key to the garage of the last house we only lived in for one month. I did research on the best way to do it, and there is none really. I thought maybe I'd pull my car into the garage like I saw my mother do when I saved her life for the first time at age eleven. Either way it was important that neither Katrina nor my daughter found me in the end. I decided on a belt. I felt as though I had no choice, and I was doing it. Finally, I had found some confidence, confident that I was going through with it.

People throw around the words, "I want to kill myself," on a bad day. Usually, it really means that one wants to feel better and kill the bad feelings. But this is a time in my life when I truly felt as though it was going to happen. I couldn't live with myself, and more than anything I believed my family, and the world was better off without me. I was waiting for the holidays to pass because I didn't want to ruin them for everyone, dealing with my death. I did not want to burden anyone. I just wanted to spare them of me.

It was moving day. We were moving back to the house we owned temporarily while I looked for work and figured this out. My son was helping me move the furniture. I was what probably seemed like whining to him about the jam I was in and how depressed I was over it. I felt hopeless, and I was leaning on him. He looked at me and was cold. He said, "You'll figure it out, you always do". One would think that would be discouraging but it triggered something in my head, and I changed my mind. I chose to fight and not give up. He saved my life that day, not realizing how close I was to giving up.

I was on damage control. We were back at the old house, living off fast food. The house was infested with mice, and we couldn't cook in the kitchen anymore because it became unsanitary, I couldn't afford an exterminator. We were using the neighbor's Wi-Fi. Trying to figure out how I was going to fix this one. The neighbors saw us move out and back a couple times and it was embarrassing. In times of need you do what you got to do though! I kept fighting.

I found a full-time job at a third-party cellphone dealer. I was making minimum wage plus commission. I worked my ass off. I was working and grateful for it. I geared up every day with make-up and Bandages to cover my tattoos and went to work. I eventually found us a small affordable, yet clean place to live. It was small but in a better neighborhood. It was a close call. Things could have gone in a totally different direction. Every decision made determines the next moment every day of our lives. I was grateful once again to be alive.

I sold three times more than anyone else, top sales month after month. I was promoted to manager of that same store within six months and then to district manager by the end of the following year. I busted my ass, luckily my back was doing much better, and I was able to. For the first time in my life, I was making six figures as a district manager. I went from almost living in my truck to minimum wage, to making six figures in one years' time. I kept the key to that old garage; I still have it. It's a reminder of the day I almost gave up.

Chapter 18

Heartache

A couple of years later, the biggest challenge I'd face was heading my way. My youngest daughter's mental health was declining rapidly. We started managing her mental health and difficult behavior since she was little. It became significant in second grade when she refused to take orders from teachers. She was attending a catholic school when the principle told me that I needed to enroll her into public school. I was told that she would have access to additional resources that they couldn't provide. It was obvious that she was very strong willed as a toddler even.

Besides school resources, we sought out professional help as well. Katrina stressed my family history which also influenced her treatment. I didn't believe in meds for a child, but my opinion was followed with allegations that I didn't want to help her. I felt guilty filling her little hand with pills.

As the years went on, the worse it became. She was bullied in school early on and it became severe in jr High and high school. She was an easy target with kids because unfortunately she would react. People got a kick out of her reactions. School became a trigger for her in the worse way. This went on for years. Unfortunately, learning became secondary for her. School was a trigger associated with struggles and anxiety.

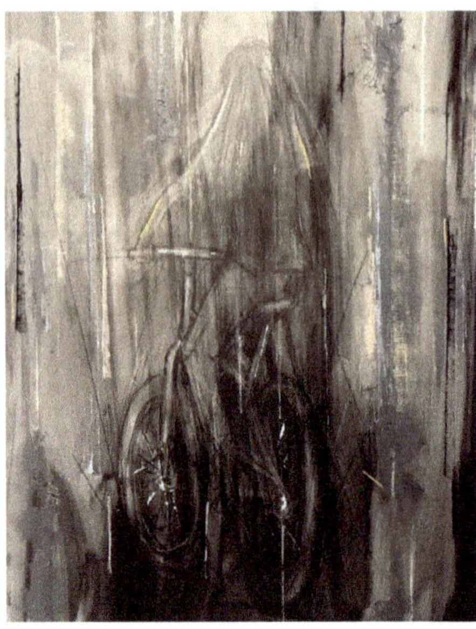

BIKE IN THE RAIN (2017)

This acrylic on canvas painting expresses a child growing and becoming independent.

I always did everything I could. I advocated for her with teachers, parents, and her own mother at times. She would call me from school often, crying. Several times a week. It became a rare day when she didn't. It was so sad. I often left work just to comfort her. She had always given her mom a hard time, they clashed. At fourteen, even myself she was starting to give a hard time to as well. The poor kid was just struggling in the worst way with her anxiety and depression. She had a difficult time processing it.

I never claimed to be perfect, there were times I could have done a better job, but honestly who can't from time to time. I put in the hard work and did my best. I was a nurturer. Her mother had a bad habit of thinking out loud, and not thinking of how her words affected other's feelings. She was more interested in getting her thoughts off her chest than communicating affective words. I failed sometimes too, but I sincerely always gave it my best. Maybe she did too. I'd rather catch a beating than have my feelings hurt by someone that is supposed to love me. We all make mistakes. The difference is when you know it and can admit it.

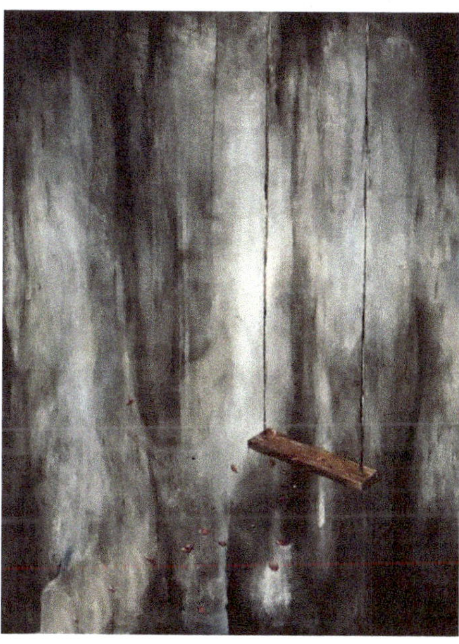

SWING BACK

(2017)

This acrylic on canvas painting expresses heartache. Rose pedals falling from an empty swing.

I've seen my daughter struggle something terrible with her depression and anxiety. So, heart breaking, I choose not to speak of the details. A good dad wants to help fix things, it's hard to accept when it's out of your hands and can't.
All I could do is be the best dad possible. Visiting her daily and being supportive when she went to the hospital and treatment centers was one of the most heart wrenching experiences of my life. She was difficult with me also at that point, but she was still closer to me than anyone else. She trusted me more than anyone and depended on me for

support. Even if I was upset, she knew I would be there for her. I was the most understanding. To be honest the treatments were making things worse. I never liked the meds. I never saw them help my mother and they were not helping my daughter much either. I didn't feel good about it.

I have always been her number one cheerleader. I have always been there to listen when she needed to talk, no matter what time of the night. I advocated for her. There was a point that things were pretty rough. I started to become in fear for her future, her life even.

It was scary when professionals seemed to start giving up and suggesting group home settings. She wasn't a bad kid. She was a teenager to start off with and that is almost always challenging itself. She lived with severe anxiety and depression. Her mom also struggled with impulse control. Being so young she had difficulties processing her emotions. Asshole kids in school didn't make it any easier for her. She just needed to be monitored carefully and we all needed to be patient while she learned self-awareness. She was just too damn young. She couldn't even tell anyone how she felt.

I always had hope, and faith. I became more depressed myself because she saved my life when my father died, filling that empty void of loss. She has always been special to me. I felt like a failure as a dad because no matter what I did, she was slipping away. When the doctors wanted to have her placed in a group home, Katrina agreed. There was no way I was going to allow that to happen. I told Katrina that if she even tried, I would leave her and take care of my daughter myself.

A group home would have made everyone's life easier but

my daughters. It wouldn't be easy for me either because I would have been constantly worried about her. It was a scary time, I was worried every moment of the day, every day. I felt as though life would crumble if I made one bad choice. I think I lost years of my life expectancy from those stressful times.

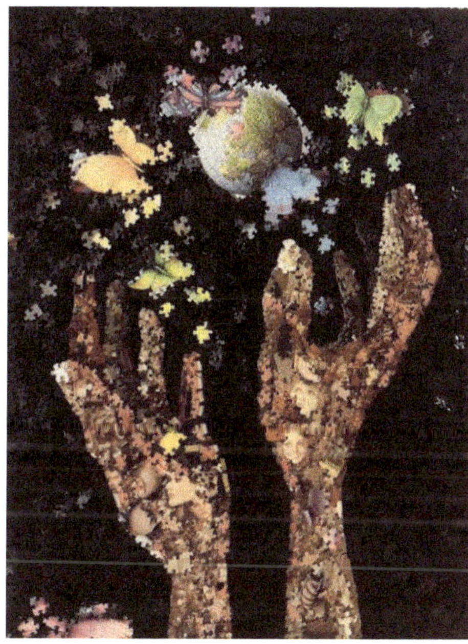

REACH

(2018)

Exploring other styles using acrylic paint, and puzzle material on canvas. This was the first puzzle composition that displays subject matter.

Things between Katrina and I were rocky, very up and down. It took its toll on our ability to tolerate each other. I know how I felt, and I know how Katrina felt because she often told me that we never should have been together, we were a bad match. She was right though, but her delivery of the messages was heartless and mean.

It was an extremely painful time. I was burying myself in the basement drinking and smoking and I was creating puzzle compositions and painting again. Most of my paintings at that time were inspired by the pain I was feeling. There was at times a dark sense of hopelessness. The battle fought and the faith for a better tomorrow are all documented in my artworks from that era.

For some unknown reason one day out of nowhere I decided to pick up the phone to make an appointment, and have my tattoos removed from my hands and neck. It was random. It was expensive, and it was extremely painful. Way worse than getting the ink itself. I had slowly stopped covering them with make-up. My boss was totally aware, and things were going great at work... Too good.

I had a great job, but when everything is going great, I beware, bad news is around the corner for sure. Whenever things are going that good, I always expect things to go bad soon. Things just didn't work like that for me. I think I was meant to struggle. For some reason I thought I should clean up my appearance in case I needed to find another job one day. Even though I had a good job, and no reason to leave.

I was struggling with my struggling daughter, and my marriage sucked. At least finances weren't an issue anymore. Then one day I received a phone call from jeff my boss. The owner of the business. He told me that he sold the business. I was finally making decent money. I had no money worries, and now I was unemployed again. Jeff was thankful for my help. I really appreciated him. He gave me opportunities when I was at my worst. He gave me a thank you gift and wrote me a check on his way out.

The new owner of the business immediately cut my pay in half and made a lot of broken promises. They hired an experienced market manager that had just been fired from the corporation side after twenty years. The business itself wasn't doing well, and he was afraid of being fired again. He literally said, "they just fired the market manager on the west coast for low numbers in his market, so I'm going to have to let you go." He sacrificed me to save his own ass and didn't hide it well. He then asked me if I wanted to resign or be fired and then gave me a date that would be my last day. I worked another week with a date to be fired hanging over my head. Talk about bad luck. I helped build this business up for the past few years, and then it was over.

I depended on unemployment and depleted every dime I had saved up in the bank. I was going to use it for a down payment on a home one day. Instead, I had to use it all to survive and provide. I had a marriage dangling by a shoestring, and a teenage daughter spiraling out of control. No one was as devoted to her well-being or sacrificed for her as I did. All with no regrets. I would have done anything to help her have a brighter future. That was my main objective.

Katrina and I drifted far from each other. I may have been the only one that realized it at first. I tried to communicate with her, I figured everything else sucked, let's try to enjoy each other more, at least. I was called selfish. I was told that I shouldn't have been wanting to enjoy life because there were so many challenges going on. I was trying to survive as a human. Otherwise, I would be useless to anyone else, never mind myself. I was belittled and I felt very insignificant. My morale, my confidence, and self-esteem was at an all-time low.

Finally, I was offered a job as a manager on the corporate end of the same company I was just working for. Tough gig but it paid the bills. It was a struggling company trying to merge with another. Sales were slow, and cramming was encouraged. Not my idea of fun, but I knew what paid the bills. I had been selling artwork online too, and it had been a while since I last did.

I was attempting to juggle and balance a life for the sake of my own sanity, but I was the only one interested in that. This cycle of trying to make the best out of each day went on for a while. I would sometimes fantasize of a day that I could go my separate way. I closed my eyes and pictured what it would be like. But I just kept accepting life for what it was. I had become so self- critical that I began to think that I was lucky that someone would want to be with me. I had no self-value. I didn't think that I had much to offer. I didn't think much of myself anymore.

I am always in an attempt to make today better than yesterday, and tomorrow better than today. It seemed like most days were a failure. I was approaching the end of my forties, and it was making me think about my own mortality. The death-bed self-reflection I would sure have one day, that we all inevitably face. I had a difficult conversation with Katrina. I told her right out that I was unhappy. For the sake of time spent, and family, I was not going to just give up.

Her reaction was not what I expected. She told me that I expected too much along with a few other belittling low blows. More hurtful were damaging things that were said including picking apart each one of my kids for their flaws and challenges, then blaming me as their bad father. Even constantly bringing up my dead mother's mental health, while throwing my past mistakes in my face to own the conversation. I had never felt so bad about myself as I did in that moment.

I just wanted to feel a bond with my partner. I was doing my best to not just give up, even though I felt the urge to do so. I sincerely tried for the sake of our daughter and the many years invested into the relationship. I didn't hate Katrina; but at that point I didn't like her anymore. We were just damaged. As always, my art told deep stories of that era.

The void between Katrina and myself became bigger. We had differences on how to handle my daughter's mental health and behavior. Katrina had stopped being physical a few years back, but she was verbally abusive in my opinion. I chose to stay though. It was my choice. I continued to create artwork, love my daughter, and push forward each day.

Experience goes far. I was older when my youngest daughter was born, and I know damn well how I wanted everything to be. I was going to see it through till the end. I'd be in her life full-time as she grew up. I raised her from the very beginning. Even when it meant sacrificing, I did what I needed to do. I can remember Katrina fighting with me, and my daughter being just a few years old. I was thinking to myself. "Ugh… X number of years left". Not anxious for her to be grown, but anxious to recover what life I had left in front of me, without losing my daughter. I didn't want her to grow up without me. I was sincere and put in the hard work.

I tried to communicate and repair the marriage. It is hard when there is bitterness and resentment involved, but I tried. I didn't really think Katrina and I separating would hurt Katrina, after all she was constantly telling me that being with me was a "big mistake." She was not interested in fixing things when I said I was unhappy. I assumed she was unhappy as well. At this point I was not my best anymore either. It was a vicious cycle, and we were caught in it. I think

Katrina was ok living like that, but I wasn't.

Katrina thought everyone needed meds, but herself. And as a result, everyone but her was medicated. If I was sad, I needed meds, if I was energetic and in a great mood, I must be manic and need meds or an increased dose. I was never fond of psych meds. I used to get sick to my stomach when putting the pills in my daughter's tiny hands daily. She was proud when she was able to gulp them down all at once with one sip of water. It became part of life for her. I don't think they even helped her at all, in fact things were worse at times. I regret allowing it to happen.

Having a bad day is normal, everyone gets sad sometimes. If things in life are sad then being sad is a normal human reaction, it doesn't always mean that you need to take medication... so you can accept terrible things. Sometimes people who take medication are not taking it for themselves, it's often taken for the people around them. So that other people can deal with you more easily at home and at work. To simply help one stay out of trouble.

I fought to keep my daughter out of a group home. All I had to do was pull the cord and say, "Okay "just once and she would have been gone. I had her on lock down though, but I wanted to let her live like a normal kid as well. I set up safety precautions to protect her from herself. I had outside around the house and common rooms inside the house equipped with cameras and sensors, except her bedroom and bathroom of course. But I had sensors on windows, so I would know if they were opened. She had GPS tracking on her phone and her bike.

I know that you can't always trust kids because kids lie too. In the moment, kids like to be left alone to do what they want. They will later think back about it one day and be disappointed. A parent taking the easy way out or letting friendship with their kid come before parenting them is not good. The child will eventually resent them for the lack of loving guidance. Deep down kids want to be guided. Being a good parent takes effort!

If that time in my life had a name, I would call it Hell. I feel like I have been through so much shit. Relatively speaking, at this point I was burnt out completely. It's not that my terrible experiences are unheard of, It's the consistency of them. I never seem to catch a break. I haven't had any peace time. It was all starting to get to me. I left home at seventeen and the struggle has never ended.

Life was daily turmoil and it always had been in one way or another. Like things weren't bad enough, Covid hit. We were all told that we might die. The stress was horrendous. Everything was closed. Makeshift hospitals were set up outside in parking lots. The country was basically in quarantine. The world was shutting down. It was unprecedented. I was lucky enough that cell phones were considered essential. I got to keep my job, when many did not. I spent each morning trying to find the essentials needed to live like toilet paper, soaps and hand sanitizer were on top of the list and the most difficult to find.

People everywhere were filled with anxiety and had a new outlook on life. Like being a person who had a close to death experience. Almost died but didn't. Although millions did die around us, the rest of us had a second chance. We were survivors of something deadly. The businesses were mostly shut down and everyone was in the house rediscovering themselves. The world was coming to a standstill, and panic was ramping up. I did a lot of painting at the time and unintentionally reflected on my own life and mortality.

I had just turned forty-eight. The thought that I was turning fifty soon was lingering in my head. I had spent a lot of my life struggling emotionally, mentally, and financially. I knew that I was probably past the halfway mark in life and the second half would end with me just getting old. I had been reaching for goals that always seemed to be right in front of me, yet out of reach.

I am a deep thinker. I thought about myself laying on my death bed one day. My daughter was approaching eighteen in a year and was showing signs of being more independent. I thought about the thoughts that I imagined would be going through my head in my final hours and minutes one inevitable day, hopefully many years away.

Asking myself if I would have regrets. Would I be at peace with whatever weight I carried on my shoulders. Would I wish I had a do over? Will I be satisfied with the efforts I put into life? Will I think I should have done something different? Will I be filled with overwhelming guilt in my final moments? Would guilt be from denying myself happiness or would it be from those that I hurt being happy? I asked myself If I would be able to die peacefully with most of my choices, at least. It will be too late to recalculate my actions then. We only get one trip across this planet in the body we were given. Once it's over, it's over. Even if we come back, we won't be this, we will be that.

I had several unsuccessful conversations with Katrina. I nearly begged her to listen. I told her that I was not happy several times, over the course of a couple of years. I could not have been clearer when I said, and I quote, “I am unhappy.” A person gets to a certain point when you feel like you are the only one trying. She took me for granted. I felt as though she believed that she deserved better than me. She was not willing to admit there was a problem and help me fix it. She just continued to say things leading me to feel as though something was wrong with me, and I felt extremely bad about myself.

We are who we are, and we don’t change much other than from the lessons we learn from life’s experiences, good and bad. I have made the best of things over the years because that is what we sometimes do as humans, we adapt and accept. I believe that is what Katrina did too. Of course, there were some good times. Everything being relative, how much of it was tolerance. I tried to make it work, and I am sure she feels that she did as well.

My forties were winding down, the pandemic gave me a new outlook as it did for many others. I started to lose weight. I lost thirty pounds without trying. I went to my doctor, and he ran a battery of tests. I waited for the results, and I was ready for the worst. Come to find out I was healthy. When I am under a lot of stress, I cannot maintain weight.

More now than ever in my life I was in touch with my own mortality. I just could not live with this being my life. I could not live with knowing I was destined to lay on my death bed one day with regrets, and guilt that I neglected myself. My one shot here on earth slipping away. I thought that there must be a way to not neglect myself and not neglect others at the same time.

It was not fair to Katrina one would think, but it was not fair to me for her to cause me to feel this way either. The number one breakdown of a relationship is failed communication and the consideration for the other's feelings, and needs. It is not easy to walk away from a twenty-year relationship, even when it's bad. Some people sometimes stay in relationships with extreme abuse simply to avoid the fear of change. Sometimes events lead a person to believe they cannot do better.

I needed to be sure that I made every effort, especially for my daughter. I communicated well and clearly. I wear my heart on my sleeve by nature, I am not capable of holding back my feelings. It did not happen overnight. It was something that had been simmering for years, addressed, and ignored.

My efforts were responded to with verbal abuse and gaslighting. I was at my breaking point. I thought, "why should I care if she doesn't." as I believed she didn't truly care. Either way I did what I do best when I am in turmoil mentally or emotionally... I paint. I was not trying to create anything. I was just allowing my emotions to move my paintbrush.

I started a new series of paintings titled Pandemic. Not because they have anything to do with the pandemic. That was just the era I created them in. As always painting was a great escape for me, a stress reliever. As always, I was painting my emotions. These paintings were inspired by my love for Picasso.

I was intrigued by his freedom with the brush. He did what he wanted to do, he thought how he wanted to think. He had the ability to truly be himself regardless of how people perceived him. Although he was criticized, being himself made him victorious. He is a legend that will never be forgotten, because he was an inventor of free-thinking art.

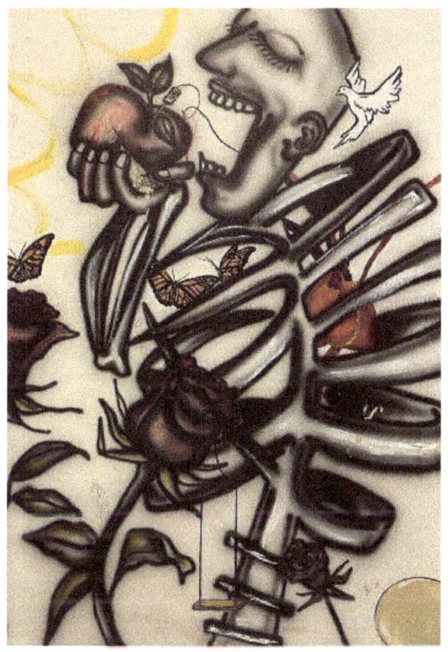

MEDICINE (2020)

This acrylic on canvas painting was a spontaneous creation that started the series titled Pandemic. There is a lot to see in this visually stimulating work of art.

Chapter 19

Facing mortality, entering my 50s

I had decided that I was going to give up on this idea of restoring the marriage. I wanted to restore my life while I still had a little time left. For the first time it hit me that my daughter was going to grow up and have her own life one day. She started dating and leaving home with friends a lot at that point. I had kept her close under close supervision for as long as I could. For the first time in many years, I had free time.

I wanted to take advantage of the little bit of youth I had left in me. I needed to find a way to make myself smile because I was dying inside. I may have seemed a little selfish, and I guess I was. Is it ever allowed? I started hobbies and spent a lot of time working on my car. Modifying it until there was nothing left that I could do to it or afford to do.

I always took care of myself physically. I knew that youth was going to slowly slip away eventually. Females were still hitting on me, and not old ladies either. I still didn't stray away at all. I was often told that I looked good for my age and cleaned up well.

With my daughter almost eighteen, she was doing her own thing more and more as teenagers do. At first, I missed her being little, but I learned to embrace the change as best I could. I just hoped to reap the reward of seeing her mature and be the best she can be. A breakup with Katrina was not going to ruin my daughter at this point. I have been giving my all to someone that considered me to be less than she deserved. At least that's what her words led me to believe.

With death knocking on my psychological doorstep, I had options. The only option I was interested in was surviving and surviving meant finding a way to smile. If I couldn't make a change I was going to fall apart, and that wouldn't be good for my daughter either. I was deeply depressed. With this extra time on my hands, I was contemplating life! Because of Covid, businesses closed down and quarantine was in full affect for weeks. There was a lot of time for thinking.

The country was shut down from the COVID pandemic. I was working once a week for a while. The stores were consolidating employees to one location until quarantine ended and we reopened all the stores again. My daughter was doing her own thing. She had a boyfriend. I painted and continued to do a lot of thinking.

I stayed in touch with the staff from my store, to check in on them. Plus, it became even more lonely for me with the world shut down. There was one girl, Nathalia, who I knew was totally alone, with her family living in a different country, so I checked on her more than the others. I enjoyed talking to her.

I started reaching out to Nathalia more often than the others. We always got along good at work and joked a lot. She had a great sense of humor and a deep thinker too. I have always loved quality conversation. The conversations were great, and they got longer, and more frequent as the days went on. Everything was still very innocent.

It got to a point where we expected to talk once nighttime came. Without meaning to we were getting to know each other very well, and we surprisingly had a lot in common. We learned that we both were miserable in the lives we had individually, and we found that we were not miserable when talking to each other. We quickly became attracted to each other, from the inside out. Even though I was planning an exit from the relationship with Katrina, this relationship forming wasn't planned.

We worked together for about a year prior. She was twenty-four years younger than me. She had an old soul, and we would have never vibed so well otherwise. The odds were against us. We unintentionally got closer. We liked each other a lot. Previously I was excited about being alone, then I became even more excited about getting closer to Nathalia.

I was never a sleep around kind of person. I was not a bad guy. I just hung on to Katrina too long. All these puzzle pieces, scenarios and circumstances were all happening at the same time. It was like the ultimate test while I was miserable, and age was knocking on my door during a life-threatening pandemic.

Quickly all I wanted to do was talk to Nathalia. She had seen me at my worst and vice versa. We knew each other for a little while already as co-workers and friends. We learned that we both had dysfunctional childhoods, and both suffered from PTSD. Both our mothers were mentally ill. We both loved art. This was huge to me. We both liked to write. We liked many of the same things, and we had similar goals.

Even before we started talking more, I was always impressed with her ability to persevere in life. She was a strong independent person, and I admired that about her. Even her willpower was extraordinary. She lost a hundred pounds over the course of two years. She didn't go on a diet or get surgery; she made lifestyle changes. She had a challenging life from a very young age and had every right to let herself be a loser, and no one would have blamed her, like myself. But she didn't! She was extraordinary.

We started off just talking on the phone for a little while, and eventually met up one day for the first time as friends and not co-workers. I remember waiting in the parking lot for her to show up. Neither of us were sure if the other would actually be there. Even though I was already planning to get a divorce, it was not final yet. That didn't sit well with Nathalia. She was a good girl, and I was a good guy, but our attraction was deep and unavoidable.

I jumped in her car, and we drove to her house. When I walked into her house for the first time, I was nervous, yet it was exciting. I looked around and thought to myself, "So this is where she lives". The first thing I noticed was that her house was very clean. We spent the afternoon together and had the time of our life. The attraction we had instantly became stronger from that point on. It was a day that we celebrate to this day as the anniversary of our love.

We quickly became best friends. We formed a trust and had a level of comfort with each other that neither of us had ever had before with anyone else. We sincerely liked each other a lot, in a short time. I had absolutely nothing to offer her other than myself. I was going through a lot at the time, and she was the only person that did not put any pressure on me at all, about anything. She took zero effort to be with from the beginning. She was the most pleasant, sweet person I had ever met in my life. We had a connection that was hard to explain. We were just uncontrollably drawn to one another. It was almost divine.

The next day I went to her house, with something to tell her. I struggled to get the words out because I was emotional and nervous. Life was very unstable at that time. She could tell I was trying to say something. She looked at me with a smile and said, “Go ahead, say it”. I looked her in the eyes and said, “I love you”. Her smile got bigger and said, “I love you too”. We were in love and weren’t sure what we were going to do next.

Regardless of how much denial Katrina was in, our relationship was over before Nathalia and I even met, but I hadn’t figured out an exit plan yet. Everything started happening so fast and unexpectedly. I was separating from Katrina, but originally, I wasn’t rushing because getting involved with someone romantically wasn’t part of the plan. Although falling in love with Nathalia was motivation to speed up, what was inevitably happening anyways. My daughter was living her life, and that made it a little easier, but not easy. I had been with Katrina for twenty years.

I don’t care how shitty a relationship is, after twenty years it’s not so easy to break away. One becomes almost institutionalized in the relationship. Petrified by the outside world around them, the unknown. I was facing life-changing decisions, once again. The future of a lot of people depended on the way I handled this. My future depended on the results of the choices I would be making. I was getting older, and his life change needed to be my last. It was a difficult time and a magical time all at once.

Ultimately, I became a happier person with Nathalia, even with the emotional struggles from the situation. I saw hope but I knew that I was not going to be able to make everyone happy. I was doing my very best to consider everything, everyone, and possible outcomes. I needed to not hurt my daughter who was still seventeen, and I needed to not hurt Nathalia who were both innocent people in this. I wanted to conflict as little un-avoidable pain as possible to Katrina. She had expressed a desire to not be with me often, so I didn't feel it would affect her too bad. Although, if it was challenging for me even though I was the one wanting to get a divorce, then it was sure to be at least a little difficult for Katrina as well. In the end I was so depressed that if I didn't continue my life changes, I may have just killed myself.

I'm terrible at being sneaky, it doesn't come naturally. My daughter was the first person to find out about Nathalia, and that certainly wasn't planned. She saw a heart emoji on my phone and knew that her mom did not send me those. She looked at me and said, "What was that? What's up?". I respected her enough to tell her the truth. I feared her possible reaction, but I told her how unexpectedly happy and in love I was. I was surprised when she said, "I'm happy for you". I seemed to have her blessing kind of, as fucked up as it all sounds.

Nathalia was uneasy, this wasn't something she did. She was trying to process that part herself. There was no stopping this from happening though. The attachment and feelings of belonging together was unstoppable. It was the first time I felt whole in a long time, if ever at all. I was smiling, I felt positive. My confidence was up. I was happy yet torn apart over how I was going to transition my life in the best way possible, causing the least amount of damage. I was bitter with Katrina, and did have a lot of resentment, but I know she couldn't help who she was, just as much as I couldn't help but to leave her.

I realized that there was no easy way anymore and that I just needed to pull the cord. I couldn't live that way. I outright told Katrina that I wanted a divorce. She instantly said it must be because of another girl. The timing was great and sucked at the same time. No matter what I could ever say, Katrina thought the only reason I wanted a divorce was because I was seeing someone else. Nothing I could ever say would help her believe the truth, which was that we were getting a divorce within the next year regardless. That sucks for Nathalia, because she deserved better than that stigma.

One thing that helped my consciousness is that I knew Katrina wasn't in love with me either. All the signs were there. Besides her saying it often, she envied what others had including better men. She didn't value me. She insulted my personality, opinions, feelings, ideas, and occasionally my appearances. The woman wished me death to my face more times than she said I love you. She repeatedly said that she wished she had never met me. Telling me that my kids were all degenerates because I was a bad father. That was the icing on the cake to be honest. What would lead me to believe that this woman loved me!

I am an artist. I had even given up my drive for art at one point because my spirit was broken, and she was ok with that. I had not had a gallery show in almost ten years. She never inspired me to create. For a person like me, that was important. When I told Katrina that she was never supportive of my art. She replied with, "I let you buy art supplies." She threw in my face on more than one occasion. "All the money wasted on art supplies and the paintings you never sold." She was also not a big fan of my work.

Maybe an artist as a husband isn't for everyone, but I was already an artist when Katrina met me. I realized that she would never do what was needed to give us both another chance at happiness being separated, before we became too old to do so. It was me that had to do it, I pulled the cord. I reminded Katrina of the countless times that she said that we should have never been together in the first place. I told her that one day she would thank me for making the difficult decisions I made. I promised her that she would be happy one day that I was making that decision. I had never been so sincere in my life at that moment as she asked me not to leave, and I left. I left Katrina, not my daughter. I would never tell my daughter who she should live with, but I knew what her choice would be.

I led Katrina to think I was staying with friends as long as I could. Still trying to spare her feelings, she did not know about Nathalia at first. I was trying to find a way to prevent inevitably upsetting Katrina as much as possible. I somehow thought that I could show Katrina that separating was the best thing without her thinking it was because of another girl. Meeting Nathalia did speed it up a little, but a separation from Katrina was happening anyways.

It was so clear to me that we didn't belong together. Katrina wasn't stupid, so I thought I could get her to see what I saw as well. After all she always said it, I just needed to convince her to act on it with me. Maybe, we could break up peacefully, co-parent and be friends. Then my daughter's friend went and told Katrina about Nathalia. That's went things became very difficult.

There was a lot going on, I needed to get away. A paintbrush and canvas weren't enough to ease the situation this time. Nathalia and I took a short vacation to New Hampshire. Up north is always peaceful. I went by my soon to be old house to get a new pair of sneakers I recently bought. I was on foot. Nathalia was picking me up nearby so we could head out on our road trip.

Katrina started following me with her car, taunting me. Slowly driving alongside, me as I walked frantically trying to get away. The further I got from her the better I felt, and it was becoming more obvious to me. Katrina yelled out at me, "She won't be there for you when they crack your chest open one day for open heart surgery." She loved throwing in my face the fact that Nathalia was younger than me. I knew her as a co-worker and friend before we ever became romantically involved. Knowing how caring she was, it upset me that Katrina said that.

In an instant I remembered how Katrina hassled me when my father was in the hospital. When I was hurt years back, I was struggling with pain, and she once looked at me in disgust and said, "Why don't you just die already." All these thoughts rapidly circling my mind, I said, "What makes me think you'll be there for me, you let your father rot in a state hospital for years until he died there." I knew it was a sore spot because she was filled with guilt over it. I was not trying to be mean; I just blew up and couldn't take it anymore. My thoughts raced rapidly. I was so frustrated and just needed her to go away and let me be.

We were losing respect for each other; I was not my best self either. A vicious spiral of disrespect started in the very beginning. Open wounds remained on both sides. I have no regrets other than the way I handled some of the situations. At this point this was all affecting my already declining mental health badly. I was doing my best at the time

It was a low blow, and I felt bad after saying it. I did apologize after that at some point. But I was just so done and needed to move on so badly. I was on the cusp of losing my fucking mind, or life for that matter. I was a ticking timebomb ready to explode and I was aware of it. Self-awareness saved me from myself.

It was not a spontaneous thing as Katrina accused me of. It had been manifesting for years, especially the last couple. I literally told her in plain English a few times within that year prior that I was terribly unhappy, and she didn't give a shit. I made efforts that she ignored. I spent a year trying to reverse the vicious spiral we had going. The marriage had been over years ago, I was just hanging on because I was used to it. Up until then I was just focused on my daughter, but now she was getting older and was not so little anymore.

I was struggling so badly that I was about to take my last breath if I stayed and tolerated this life any longer. I couldn't get away fast enough. I felt as though I was going to burst. I honestly felt as though this was my last chance at happiness. After how life had gone thus far. Only I can make me happy, but only the person you are with can provide the environment you need to be the best person you can be.

After that statement about her dad, Katrina drove away and left me alone. I was able to move on with the day. I felt bad because I know I hurt her feelings. I was so built up with frustration. To fight the guilt, I would think about the things she had said to hurt me in the past, and that helped.

Nathalia and I drove to New Hampshire. It was magical. It was a time we will never forget. On the way there it was raining, and we stopped at a Walmart up there. We were standing in the parking lot holding an umbrella with the company logo on it from the place we were working when we first met. We were also wearing face masks because we were deep into the COVID pandemic at that time, and face masks were required everywhere we went.

We took a picture there that day in the parking lot that will always be an iconic moment for us. It clearly displays an important moment in our history. I later painted that picture for her on canvas. The picture tells a story of love and struggle. We had been going through a lot of emotional strain, and this time away together was exactly what we needed to clear our heads.

When I got back, I dreaded dealing with Katrina, but it was not avoidable. She immediately started manipulating me and making me think I was going crazy. Katrina just could not imagine how I would want to leave her unless I was crazy. She obviously was not paying attention to me at all. I was extremely overwhelmed; I did not intend to hurt anyone.

I told her that there was nothing wrong with her, or me. We were not meant to be together, as she had said herself many times before. It was time we made a move. I just wanted everyone to be happy, Katrina included. She instantly went for my soft spot; she went for my daughter and convinced her that I was a horrible person and Nathalia must have been manipulating me. She even went as far as to suggest that she was using Voodoo to trap me.

I am a compassionate person, to the point of self-destruction at times. I thought to myself, maybe I was crazy and manic like I was being told. Maybe I would regret it after. Maybe the grass isn't greener, and maybe it's me, like Katrina has been saying this whole time. I was starting to think that I might be going crazy, like my mother did. Katrina kept telling me that I should be lucky to have someone that wants me even though I have all these problems. This was being drilled into me daily. Messing with my thought process and telling me how sick I am. I started having trouble thinking for myself.

I became afraid because I was possibly manic and out of control but didn't see it. I was so torn between being with Nathalia, someone that I believed was perfect for me and that made me happy versus doing what was expected of me. At this point I was starting to lose it a little. The pressures of life-changing choices were overwhelming. My daughter was being told that I was a terrible person, and that made it even harder. She was starting to believe her mom and started giving me a hard time. She went from being happy for me to being angry with me.

My daughter still wanted to live with me though. Her mother also wanted her with me too. Katrina seemed to only be concerned about herself, as she called me narcissistic. Throughout this time Katrina kept expressing the amount of time we had been together and the change in lifestyle she would endure from a break-up. She even offered me an open marriage if I stayed just to help with the bills. That just validated my decision. Someone that loves you doesn't make that negotiation. A scenario like that is based on convenience.

I was getting angry with Katrina, she wouldn't admit seeing what I saw, which she had said herself so many times prior. Now our daughter was old enough for us to make a change that would give us both a second chance at life, and Katrina was making it so damn hard. It eventually got ugly between us for a while.

I did not expect Katrina to be happy about my choices. But I didn't expect to be in for what I had ahead of me. I had made it clear that the marriage was over before Nathalia came into the picture and that was the truth. I was leaving her and planning my transition for some time. I also understand why Katrina found it hard to believe, but I couldn't change that. It sounds like I was trying to not be the bad guy. That wasn't true, I just wanted the truth to be known. I knew no matter what I said, I would always be the bad guy in this story though.

With Nathalia I felt appreciated for who I was, and it was euphoric. She showed me what it felt like to be good enough. It was beyond being just the honeymoon period. We knew how real it was. We knew the best and worst qualities each had and appreciated how those things made us the people each other loved. I recall when I literally looked up at the sky and thanked God for putting her in my life. I had spent so much time suffering in my life from disappointment and traumas. Here I was with everything I have ever needed right in front of me.

I struggled in my head because I was still being manipulated by biased people telling me that I was Manic, out of my mind for doing what I was doing. Constantly comparing me to my mother. If she was sick, I must have been too. People thought that I must have been crazy to walk away from a long-term relationship, not thinking about how bad it must have been to cause that to happen in the first place. These things don't happen overnight, or for nothing. I wasn't a cheater; I was a human being, trying to gain better quality of life... emotionally, but at what cost to others. Guilt set in.

I was confused and I began to not trust myself. I was afraid to mess up Nathalia with my bullshit in the meantime. I was afraid of stringing her along as I didn't know if I was coming or going, mentally. She was young, she was a sweetheart. A genuinely nice person. I didn't want to ruin her too. I felt terrible, but I left her house to figure out what was the right thing to do for everyone. I was not thinking of just myself as many probably thought. It was extremely difficult to do, after all she was a dream come true.

It was crucial for me that I knew what I was doing before I dragged an innocent bystander down with me. I knew how I felt about her, I was in love. I was not totally confident in my own mind though; I became afraid of myself. Most didn't allow me to do my own thinking, and it was fucking with me big time. If I didn't go through whatever process that was ahead of me, I was afraid that I would question my actions later, and that could have been life threatening to myself. This needed to be without doubt, or I would have possibly tortured myself with what-ifs for the rest of my life. Even though I knew I was no doubt in love with Nathalia.

I admitted myself into the hospital. It was during COVID so there were no visits allowed, which was helpful in clearing my head. I would get calls from Katrina and Nathalia every day. I was always excited when she called. I would walk into my room and see a note saying, "Call Nathalia", with her number written on a post-it. Yet I was filled with anxiety when Katrina called.

Katrina and I could never speak without there being tension. That was a clear-cut sign to me. I even avoided some calls. She often started fighting with me on the phone and made me feel like shit every day. She continued to taunt me, even though I was in the hospital trying to feel better. She was angry and wouldn't let go. She took time on each call to remind me how unstable I was, and how I needed to listen to her. She took time to remind me that I was a terrible person. She didn't want to hear about what brought us to that situation. I went to the hospital because Katrina led me to believe I was going crazy, but that hospital stay helped me see the truth.

The hospital put me on a unit with extremely disturbed people for some reason. My first night sleep was terrible. My roommate kept me up all night. I told the staff that he seemed like a nice guy and all, but I couldn't stay in that room anymore. All day long he was talking to the walls. They weren't pleasant conversations either. They were violent conversations. He was talking to gang members, the mafia, and negotiating with other criminals. Then he held a conversation with God all night.

He tucked himself in and was staring up talking to the ceiling all night. I must admit, I was a little uneasy, and concerned about sleeping in there with him. The staff did room checks every fifteen minutes, but you can kill a man in less time than that. The worst part was that the bathroom didn't have any locks or real doors. They looked like old Wild West double swinging saloon doors with a space at the bottom and a space at the top. I put my sneakers at the bottom of the door, so that he knew I was in there. Trying to take a poop was a challenge.

They moved me to another unit the next day. The therapist told me I had a good reason to feel the way I did. I have been through a lot in my life. The consensus was that I was suffering with PTSD. I was dealing with severe depression and anxiety. Mood swings and self-loathing.

The only person that wasn't feeding me advice or ideas was Nathalia. She never tried to talk me into feeling any certain way. She always told me to do whatever I thought was best for me, and she would support that. She said that my happiness was all that was important at that time. This was another clearcut sign of who I wanted and needed in my life.

I left the hospital as soon as I could, and nobody knew. I bought roses and drove to Nathalia's house. I waited outside for her to arrive home from work and was so excited to see her. As she approached the house, I turned the corner to surprise her. Her face lit up with happiness, and I was just as happy to see her. It was a special moment.

The manipulation from Katrina continued instantly, soon as she knew I was out. I was made to feel like I was a selfish and bad person. My daughter was becoming tough on me too, after hearing how awful a person I was from her mother. Katrina was in fear of being alone financially. Loading me with guilt, I was made to feel like I was a horrible person for making my life important to me. I was called narcissistic. It didn't take much to persuade me into self-loathing once again. I began to believe that I didn't have the right to think I deserved happiness.

I was fresh out of the hospital and still healing. I left Nathalia's house again, I left things behind this time because I knew I would be back, I just had to figure this out. Katrina turning my daughter against me was making it hard. I was trying to be happy and not have anyone upset with me for it. I guess that was going to be impossible, and I would soon see that.

I forced myself to do something that I truly didn't want to do. I spent most of my time alone, working on my car, keeping myself occupied. My daughter had a boyfriend and was doing her own thing. I painted a bunch to pass the time. I couldn't stop thinking about Nathalia. I missed her dearly. I kept picturing her face in my mind. Visualizing her facial expressions and reminiscing about our conversations. One thing about her that was different than anyone else is that she allowed me the time to process everything and do what I needed to do. I know it wasn't easy for her, but she had faith and patience.

One afternoon I found out that the dog Nathalia adopted finally arrived from Georgia. As soon as she opened the cage, the dog ran away into the woods. I felt so bad because I had already been putting her through so much, and now this happened to her too. I felt terrible and I knew that she needed me, so I drove to Boston and met up with her. We were searching for her dog at an old cemetery all afternoon without success. It was getting dark, and we couldn't see anymore. I had a long drive back, and it wasn't easy to leave Nathalia behind.

I emotionally hit rock bottom. I went home to Katrina's house and was deeply, hopelessly depressed. I felt like I ruined everyone's life, Nathalia, Katrina, and my daughter's life. I already carried guilt over feeling like I abandon my mother and father, to later be left to call the shots on their death. My brother, my sister, Jr., Tammy, who I could have done more for. Even Jimmy, If I helped him instead of abandoning him years before that, maybe he wouldn't have become a drug addict.

Katrina found me before it was too late. I had passed out with a rope tied snug around my neck. She was totally disgusted with me, yelled at me, and walked away. She showed no compassion. I was so broken. I wanted to be with Nathalia. Katrina was continuing to tear me down, and now my daughter was looking down at me for the first time too. It was beginning to be too much.

I went for treatment, spent some time away from everyone. I was back in the house that Katrina lived in. A short time had gone by, and I was convinced that there was no way I could stay with Katrina, nor was I going to be able to stay away from Nathalia. I was stuck.

I became a puppet jacked up on Lithium and a bunch of other stuff. I was a zombie, and my creativity also became extremely challenged. I even agreed to try marriage counseling with Katrina, at her request. It just wasn't going to work, especially with the daily reminders of how much of an awful person I was. The guy spent the entire forty-five minutes putting me down, and never discussed the root causes. I was torturing myself, and it was becoming clearer and more definite that I wanted to be with Nathalia.

Katrina and I had been over for a while, and we were beating a dead horse to death. If something didn't change, it was all going to be the death of me. I killed a lot of time working on my car. One morning I couldn't help myself. I reached out to Nathalia and told her that I missed her. I told her that it was obvious that I was never gonna be able to go on without her. I didn't know how to do it, but I needed to be with her. We met up the next day. We were so excited to see each other we just talked and talked and talked.

I know she was hurt during some of that process, and I will forever feel bad about that. She didn't deserve it. It had to happen for her to get the best version of me... forever. It was never about me questioning my love for her. She had faith, and I did too. The fact that she never tried to persuade me, or even allow me to feel guilt was huge. I felt no anxiety or pressure from her. It was so liberating. She was a unicorn. Absolutely amazing and fell into my life at just the right time. I was the luckiest man alive to have her, and it was obvious.

She was just happy to be with me, and it showed. As I felt the same as well. I had never seen such a happy soul. That drew me even closer to her. She cared about me and wanted me to be happy at any cost. Me being so broken, I was already a mess. She still loved me for me and who I was. She believed in me, and I really needed that.

Nathalia also accepted my daughter with open arms and showed her positivity. That was very important. She quickly became a positive role model. My daughter didn't make it easy for her either. I didn't have to second guess what I said, or criticize myself anymore., Nathalia somehow convinced me that I was special and helped me see the good things about myself and be proud of who I am, instead of being disappointed in myself.

If I laid my head on my pillow one night to sleep, and then woke up in the morning to find out It was all a dream, it would have been so sad. I would not have been surprised though; it would have made sense. Because I had never had anyone treat me so well before. In every other past relationship, they wanted to change me into their idea of acceptable. Nathalia loved me for who I was.

There was no keeping us apart. I was one hundred percent convinced of what I wanted to do. The next day we met at Roger Williams Park. I remember it like it was yesterday. I was so excited on the drive there. As I approached her, she looked like an angel standing there with the sun shining through her blonde hair. I looked closer and tucked inside her overalls was a little dog. Her name was Hope. She was named Hope because she was the only one that survived the delivery, including her mom. She was an Italian Grey Hound, and she was now our dog.

Hope was a replacement for the one that ran away. Nathalia knew that I wanted an Italian Greyhound after seeing her friend's. Hope had some trauma issues that we soon learned. It took a while before she trusted anyone except Nathalia. Eventually I won her over too by earning her trust.

From that day on we met every morning and went for a walk and just talked. We just wanted to be together. Trying to figure out how we were going to make this happen, while inflicting as little pain as possible to others around us. One thing for sure was that I wasn't letting Nathalia go this time. I finished processing. I wasn't going to let this one God given chance at happiness pass me by, plus I cared about her very much. It was truly magical. We were so much in love and still are today.

Once again, I wasn't good at sneaking around. It was discovered shortly after. I wasn't sneaking to have my cake and eat it too. I was sneaking because I was trying to not hurt feelings. Katrina saw a message on my phone when I fell to sleep one night. She obviously became upset to say the least and signed herself into the hospital herself. I toggled between the house where my daughter was and Nathalia's house. We were obviously going to get a divorce at this point. My effort to help Katrina realize that we didn't belong together failed.

Katrina left the hospital and was already dating, which I was happy about. It validated when I said it was for the best. Plus, I knew she would move on quickly, and she did. She tried to keep it a secret because she wanted to keep me staying the bad guy. She was also planning what would be an extensive divorce-court battle. Getting revenge became her main objective. She consistently expressed fears of being alone and the financial repercussions from a divorce.

Chapter 20

Self-Discovery

My daughter and I went to stay with Nathalia. My daughter was a little confused with the info she was being fed from the other side, but deep down she loved me and did like Nathalia. She also knew what I went through in the relationship with her mother. I was very grateful that she was so good to my daughter, that was an important piece to this. She was still at the tail end of being a teenager and was a challenge at times still. Nathalia had the patience of an angel. They were getting to know each other. This was a process as well.

Nathalia was half my age. I was young hearted, and she was an old soul. The chances of us meeting up and being together was a long shot. Her mother became pregnant with her after she crossed the southern border by foot. She was her mom's first child born in the United States. Her dad brought the family back to South America when she was a little kid. He took their passports and abandoned them there. Nathalia raised her two little brothers while helping care for her mentally unstable mother. They lived in a garage until

Nathalia found work. She was in a third world country, holding on to the dream of returning to America. This matured her quickly.

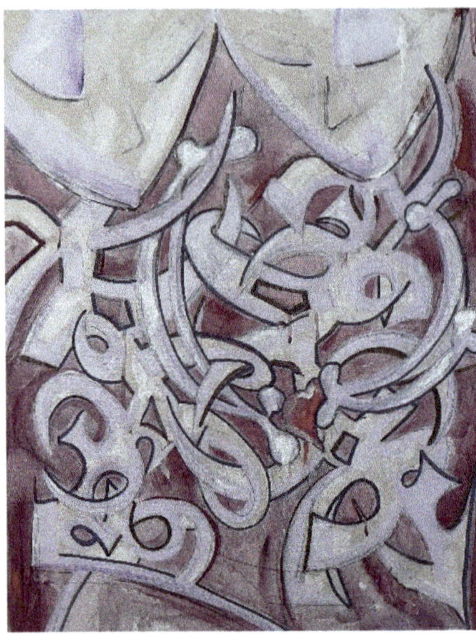

ONE HEART
(2022)

This acrylic on canvas painting expresses a mood that is seen differently depending on the viewer and their state of mind.

Everything we had gone through in life made her who she was, and me who I was. Anyone that knew us knew that our relationship was magical. She was the sweetest person I had ever met in my life. A very likable person. She put in the effort too to bond with my daughter. She showed her that no obstacles would hold her back unless she allowed it to. My daughter even said one day, “If Nathalia did it, I can do it too”. She inspired positivity in my daughter’s life, as well as mine.

Nathalia‘s apartment was in Fall River. Natahlia welcomed my daughter to invite friends, and even went to pick them up for her, and they had a good time. She fed them all and even brought them home the following day. It was still a far drive from where my daughter was used to living, so she went back to her mom’s house temporarily. It didn’t last long before

Katrina was calling me daily complaining. She wanted my daughter back with me as soon as possible because she was giving her a hard time. Katrina was being aggressive and persistent, giving me deadlines. She gave me thirty days to find an apartment closer to her because that is when my daughter was planning to come back with me.

Nathalia and I rushed to find a place that was big enough for all three of us, and not too far from where my daughter was used to living, for convenience. Trying not to disturb her life too much. It was a challenge to say the least.

Nathalia didn't have any credit and my credit was shot by the whole situation that had just taken place. I maxed out my credit cards by the time the dust had settled. Luckily, Nathalia came across this nice one-family house on a dead-end street. Seemed like something we would never get.

I was still paying Katrinas rent for months while not living there, as well as her car insurance and cellphone bill. I wanted to help her and give her a chance to save some money. That meant that Nathalia and I didn't have much money saved. We were living on prayers at that time.

We met the property owners, and a few days later they approved us. We had a nice home to live in. Nicer than anything either of us had ever lived before. Moving day was hell yet refreshing. It was a fresh start. We moved two apartments into one house in just one day. It was one of the most physically exerting days of my life. Motivated by hope and love.

My daughter was confused. Even though she wasn't very close to her mother at that time, her parents split up and life was changing. On top of that she was having boyfriend issues. Katrina didn't help much when she made every effort to crush my reputation in revenge. She said terrible things about Nathalia and me to her. Some people were more interested in hurting me than helping a child get through her own challenging times. I tried my best to filter what I said, but it was hard when I needed to defend my integrity against biased opinions and exaggerated facts.

My daughter became difficult to live with. I secluded myself away in the same house, to avoid conflict. It only made matters worse until one day there was a big blow out and she went to stay with her mother. She came at me as I was having a bad day, and the situation escalated. It was the first time we argued in a while. She was hurtful in the things she said, using her mouth as a sword.

She went to live with her mother again. To be fair she was a teenage girl, and one would think that her mom would be an important person at that time in her life anyways. I was trying to heal from I don't even know what I just went through and still was. I couldn't be there for her or anyone else if I wasn't stable myself. Even though I had met the love of my life, I was still a broken person trying to heal.

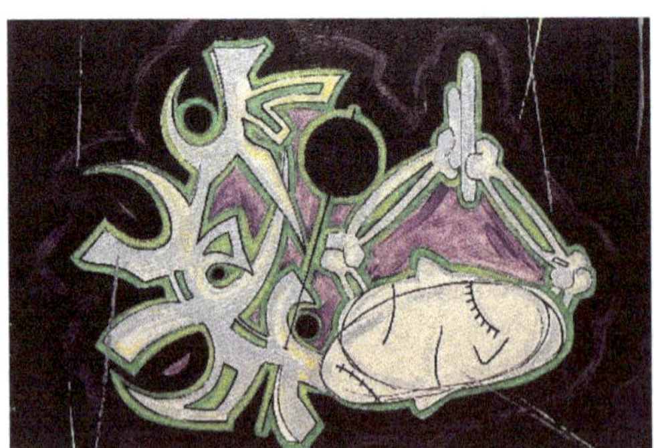

MERCIFUL
(2021)

Acrylic on canvas painting. Praying for a better tomorrow.

It had been a few weeks, and I hadn't heard from my

daughter, and I couldn't get her to reply. I made a video slideshow with pictures of her and myself, from over the years. I attached the song, Just the Two of us. She ignored it and every other attempt I made to make things better. I still thought she was supervised a little and safe at her mom's. I was not aware of what was actually happening.

My daughter was angry with me, and that was crushing. I tried to reach out to her a few times but was rejected. I didn't want to lose communication for so long that it would become awkward. I wanted her to say sorry, as petty as it seemed to her, but she wouldn't. To me that admission of being wrong would show that she acknowledged what she did and will try not to repeat it again. How else could we ever get past it so we could live in harmony.

She was hurtful in things she had said. She and her mother became a fighting force against me for a few months, and that hurt badly. Her mother won that battle. I lost my daughter for a short time, which was extremely hurtful.

A few months later when she eventually asked to move back in, she was handling it wrong. Her attitude was terrible, and I knew that things were sure to get bad again and fast. She needed to learn how to respect me. It was one of the hardest things I ever did, but I said, "No". I had always been there for her, so it was a shock to her. I told her that I could not handle the aggression from her at that time.

I was fighting my own demons with challenged mental health. I may have seemed selfish, but I was just trying to survive. Trying to get through it all without making mistakes. Not long before that, I was rocking on the edge of existing or not. I choose to give it my best. That meant me being a little selfish for a short time. Anyone that truly loved me should have been able to understand that.

The number one thing that I needed to fight for was my mental health and self-awareness. I had to find myself before I could be there for my daughter or anyone else. Nathalia was supportive and gave me zero stress. My daughter turned eighteen and she had her mother as well. I should have been able to take that time to heal. I could tell by our conversations that she wasn't ready yet. All I wanted was respect.

Little did I know she was barely even with her mother. Katrina wasn't being supportive and drove her away. My daughter was now walking down a dark path with people she had met in that short time. Drug addicts, gang members and other dangerous people in other dangerous situations that I didn't find out about for a little while.

If she didn't want her there, she could have used her head and stopped making me out to be a villain, so my daughter wouldn't be giving me such a hard time. I was paying child support for my eighteen-year-old daughter and the only people in the house were Katrina and her new boyfriend. I wasn't aware but my eighteen-year-old was barely there and about to destroy her life.

My daughter had had enough, broke down and finally called Nathalia one afternoon while I was at work and apologized. She wanted to be picked up. She and her mom were fighting badly, and her mother was being verbally cruel to her. I'm sure my daughter was a handful, but that was nothing new. The verbal abuse was extreme. It had become clear that Katrina was overwhelmed and was hurting my daughter emotionally. She and her mother were in a vicious cycle of hatred, and it was ruining my daughter. Nathalia accepted her apology, drove to her and brought her back home with us.

I wasn't truly aware of how bad it was until the tail end of it. It was a sad time to say the least. I didn't know this was all happening. I wanted her back home with me, but I was waiting for her to "Get it". So, she could come home for good, and we wouldn't have any more issues. I thought she was living with her mother the whole time. I expected her mother to be able to handle her for just a little while.

There were a few hurdles, but we all spent the next few months learning how to live together. The nine-month separation was hurtful to me and my daughter in different ways, but it created a newfound respect for each other. She saw that we were sincere and cared about her. Our environment was peaceful and positive. She was able to rest her mind and work on finding herself. We learned to respect each other as adults. It gave us time to learn how important the other was. It was like a new beginning. I wasn't just her dad anymore; I was also a human being now.

Katrina and I finally got the divorce settled legally in court. It took a while because Katrina wanted me to give her alimony, so there was a court battle. I didn't earn that much more than Katrina and we both had a lot of bills. Our child was grown, and we owned nothing significant. I originally paid her rent, Tv, cellphone and car insurance for months after I left to help her get a head start. I paid her car insurance and cellphone bill for over a year. It didn't matter because she still complained that I left her stranded even though I didn't go without helping her.

Chapter 21

Real Life

I had Nathalia who loved me, and she showed me that every day. I loved her back equally. We knew each other well and appreciated who the other was, and we still do today. My youngest daughter transitioned nicely into an adult over the past couple of years. She graduated high school and learned how to handle relationships better from her experiences. The key was self-awareness. All the hard work paid off. I set the stage allowing her to be her and be self-sufficient. We lived in a great environment, in harmony. We wouldn't have had that without Nathalia.

Nathalia and I had a bond from day one. One of us will think about something and then in a moment the other begins to talk about it. Not knowing the other was thinking about it. She is like a female version of myself. In just the first couple of years we did more than most, spending as much time together as humanly possible, and still do. Wanting to schedule our days-off together; we have truly always been best friends.

We have thousands of photos, and each anniversary I print up a summary of our year together at a glance and put it in a photo album for her, for us. We have collections of memorabilia like our coffee cup collections from all the places we've gone. We are that couple that shares a lemonade. We have loved going for walks and still do it as often as possible. Every day I feel like I love her more than the day before and it couldn't get any stronger. The next day comes, and I love her more than yesterday.

Nathalia and I went and visited MOMA in New York city, which was so exciting. We saw so many precious masterpieces that I have only seen in books, like Starry Nights, which is surprisingly fairly small. We walked into a huge room and hanging there on the wall bigger than life was the painting titled, "Dance", by Henri Matisse. We both walked into the room together slowly in awe, as tears ran down our faces simultaneously. I was a lucky man already, but in that moment, I realized how lucky I truly was to have Nathalia and still am.

I started painting more, and was engaged in my art, and Nathalia has always been very supportive and my biggest fan. She always truly believed in me, even when I didn't so much. Life was going great! The static had cleared, and we were living peacefully.

Then I woke up one morning, swung my legs off the bed to stand up. I stood on my two feet like I did every morning, except this time it was different. I felt a level of pain that I had never felt before in my life. There was a crushing feeling at the bottom of my spine that ran through my hip and down my leg. It became worse and worse as the days went on. The store I was working in closed and I was left to handle it alone and hurt myself. I pushed myself and continued to go to work and kept doing the things that I normally did.

I was petrified because I didn't want to end up ruining our financial stability. So, I continued until I couldn't do anything anymore. My boss told me I needed to take a leave because it was affecting my performance and attendance. Within a month I had lost my ability to do almost everything. It was the most painful thing I had ever felt in my life.

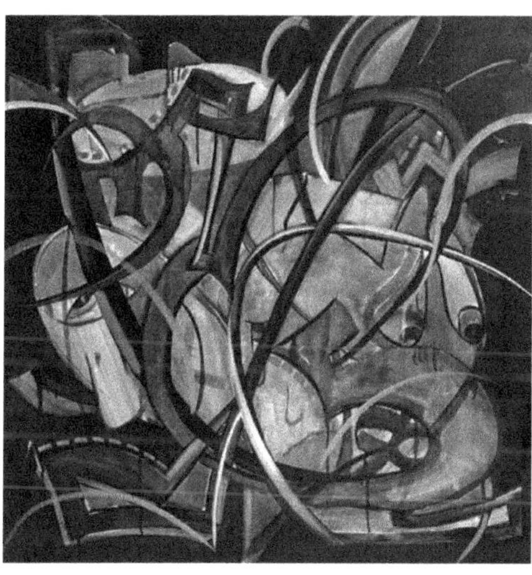

SCIATICA 1
(2022)

This acrylic on canvas painting is a visual of chronic pain, created over time, while enduring severe pain myself.

I had a sciatica flare up from a herniated disc. It took away my ability to do simple things like sit down and eat a meal yet standing hurt too. The pain started in my lower back and went through my hip and down my left leg to my foot. I needed to lay down in awkward positions for the slightest bit of relief. Taking six to eight hot showers a day to mask the pain. Watching the clock and waiting for the next opportunity to take another dose of my pain meds. I tried every cream you can imagine. I bought an inversion table, back adjuster, and every vibrating heat pad and cool pack I could find.

It was scary and excruciating. Having severe pain twenty-four-seven became traumatizing. I was out of work for months. I had to stop taking Lithium for the first time in years because the pain was so bad I needed to take ibuprofen, which I couldn't safely mix with Lithium. I pushed myself to stay active as much as I could, although I was often laid out on my back.

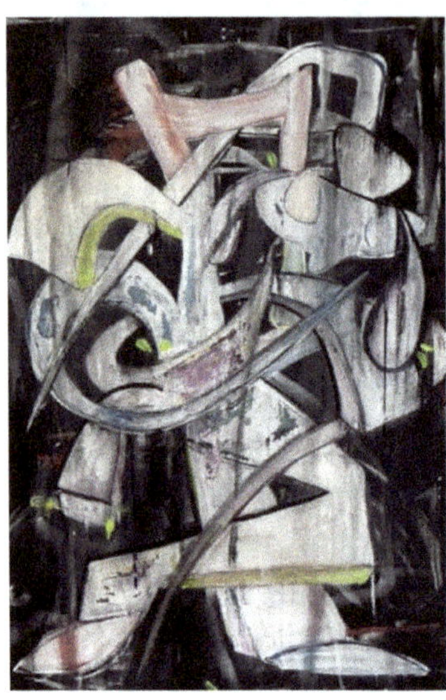

SCIATICA 3
(2022)

This acrylic on canvas painting is the third painting in a three-part series of paintings displaying a visual of chronic pain. This painting was created while in excruciating pain.

Nathalia helped me dress and shower, then head out for a full day at work. She came home and cleaned, did laundry, cooked and continued to care for me. I was absolutely useless. She never complained and never made me feel bad about myself. In fact, she went out of her way to find positive reassuring things to say to me. Always trying to lift my spirits and give me hope. She was the only person that ever helped, or even asked how I was feeling. We were not married, and she had every reason to run for the hills. I was not testing her, but God did. We were both being tested at that time.

My tolerance for pain had become strong as time went on.

Having just a little pain was a relief because it was never totally gone. Pain meds allowed a little time with less pain, and that was the only time I'd be able to paint. It was difficult to accept, I was always so active before this happened.

This period in my life was just another unexpected part of my journey. This too was life changing and a true test. More than not, a flare up will subside in a few weeks to months. I would wake up day after day wondering if it would be any better. I'd swing my legs off the bed slowly to stand up and the pain would shoot through my body, every single day, and was getting worse. I was scared for the future, but grateful that I had someone who cared and was willing to help me.

I believe that things happen for a reason. I have learned something from each fall I took in life. Between being in excruciating pain, following the near-death experience we all had with the Pandemic. All, right around the ripe age of fifty. I gathered a life full of experiences and organized my thoughts. Thinking and thinking, discovering a whole new understanding of myself. The pain was humbling.

I was out of work for almost a year, luckily my employer held my job. I was feeling some improvement and I wanted to return to work. I figured that I would be able to do it if I had reasonable help. I called my boss asking him if he would please keep me in one of the many close by locations because the driving position could be extremely painful more than often. So, they decided to graciously place me almost an hour from my home, which was the total opposite of what I requested. I pleaded and explained my reasoning. I was still healing, and I knew that I needed to avoid starting my workday off in more pain than necessary. It was crucial in my continued recovery. I was told that the transfer was what was best for my development, which was a management manipulative tactic.

I had been with the company for many years and knew how things worked. I realized that they were giving me a hard time. I expressed my observations to HR that I was being discriminated against due to my medical condition. The upper management ran the business like a football team, and I was benched, and useless to them. Within weeks I received a phone call offering me a location closer to home, and I went back with a clear accommodations request from my orthopedic surgeon. He was one of many doctors and physical therapists I had been seeing. No working more than forty hours / eight hours or less at a time, no bending, lifting, climbing, or crawling etc. The usual for a person recovering from a back injury.

Soon as I returned my new district manager met with me to discuss his requirements which included performing operations that went against my accommodation request. He stated that he would sit and go over the accommodations with me once it was approved. He also made me aware that I was losing staff including the assistant manager who would have been the one helping me. The previous manager was around but focused on a new location she was opening.

My accommodations were accepted and approved my human resources, but my district manager never had that follow up conversation. He never recognized them or implemented any procedures for me. In fact, never spoke of the accommodations again. I had little choice but to do what the job required, including the physical task and working double shifts at times. Within a few months I was in pain worse than ever. It weakened me as symptoms became worse, I acquired new additional back problems. This put me back out of work once again. I still live with pain every day my life, but it allows some well needed time to rest my mind though.

Chapter 22

Closing epilogue

It has been a while now since my back and the sciatica altered my life. I had a lot of time to reflect, and I learned a lot about myself. We all see a different version of ourselves than others see. I think of how I could have done better in certain situations. It's common to think that way, especially when someone passes away. Thinking, "If I knew sooner what I know now, I'd do things so much differently." The fact is, I needed to go through every challenging time I've had in order to be the person that I am today.

The fact is that I needed to make the mistakes I made and go through the traumas endured to become the person that I am today. I became the person that Nathalia loves, and the person that my children know they can trust and go to for solid advice and love. Everything we experience makes us who we are, good and bad. Making mistakes is how I learn how to be successful, and success looks different to everyone.

Unfortunately, bad times tend to weigh heavily on me, like most people, and it's hard to forget some things. That's the curse of being human, the most intelligent species on earth. Sometimes, you need to squint your eyes to see the good times. I believe in Karma, good and bad. Not that I think it is divine, or magical. I believe we set the stage for what happens next in our lives... usually.

If I believe in something strong enough and put in enough effort, things will work out in some way. Things working out don't always look like what we think it will either. I have learned to accept that. At this point I also accept that anything is possible. As the old saying goes, God helps those who help themselves. I believe in God one hundred percent. I think we are just not capable of understanding everything. That's where the faith comes in.

I know in my heart that there is something amazing that we just don't understand fully. We humans aren't as smart as we would like to think we are. When I pray, I don't ask God to give me things in greed. I pray more for others than myself. I ask for forgiveness, safety, and stability. I thank the lord for what I have thus far and to help me be the best version of myself each day. Maybe ask him to pave the way for me a bit and show me guidance.

Through life's experiences I grew to understand my parents more. This was a big part of healing. Kids put too much pressure on their parents, not realizing they are only human too. I wish I understood better when they were still alive. They put me through private school because they wanted me to have the best education. I was born with my feet pointed at three and nine o'clock, and my parents made sure they were fixed. My adult teeth grew in and all over the place and they got me braces that they couldn't afford. Those three things were enough to earn forgiveness from me for any bad choice they ever made. Even if a few messed me up.

Who am I to expect my parents to be perfect. I see now how much of a challenge life is, and they were only people too. Dealing with their own childhood traumas and life's curveballs themselves. Trying to make life work. Even though I shared some dark times, there were good times too, but I couldn't really see that until I grew up and had a better understanding of life. I remember laughing with my mother and joking around. I had great times with my dad going places like feeding the ducks when I was little. As a family we went to beaches and amusement parks in the summer.

I think back to some of those moments, and I can visualize them in full color. Wishing I could have a moment with my mother and father once again. Now they are gone. One day my children will hopefully do the same when I am gone one day too. I hope they will think back and cherish the little moments that they had with me too. I was the only child that my parents raised together from the beginning and all the way through. With my siblings popping in and out, I was almost like an only child, but wasn't.

My dad's passing will forever be extremely painful. I will forever be scarred by both of my parents' sudden deaths, revival and watching their eyes involuntarily open and close, day after day. Wondering if they would wake up. In the end it was my responsibility of having their life support removed. One after the other.

I have had mixed feelings about my mother over the years. Her actions started my life off on a rough path, but I learned to understand her better. I wish she was still alive to experience the great son I could be and would be to her today if she were still here. I feel like I didn't abandon her as most did, even though I understand why it happened. Even still, a part of me feels that I could have done just a little bit more to improve her quality of life after my father died. The truth is that I wasn't capable mentally of doing any better than I did.

I did the best I could do without sacrificing my own mental health completely. I was there every day off for a while until she was used to living alone. After a while when she became used to it, I picked her up some Sundays and holidays etc. She got to enjoy having grandchildren a little including her youngest grandchild until she was five.

I was so broken from childhood traumas; I was infatuated with being loved. I spent my life in bad relationships doing shit that I figured was next in life and dreaming of being the artist that God intended me to be. I had mimicked who I thought I should have been for others, almost to death. The relationships I had were not with bad people, they were with people that were wonderful for someone else, just not me.

Rhonda and I were just kids and I understand why things didn't last between us. Although the situation really fucked me up. Jess entered my life at a crucial time redirecting my path to a better place that I am thankful for. I once felt guilty for selfishly turning Katrinas life upside down for the sake of my own happiness. I felt bad because I always knew deep down that we weren't going to last, but I hung on for my daughter's sake. I think she hung on afraid of the unknown. That left Katrina alone at forty. I was sincere when I told her that she would thank me one day, but she didn't see that then of course. She met a more compatible person. Yet, she was still full of anger, even though the choice I made saved us both from lying on a hospital bed one day old, with regrets. Guilt was not necessary, I once saved her life many years ago, and I saved both our lives in the end.

In past relationship they were all cutting themselves short as well until cords were cut. No relationship is a waste of time though. They are all learning experiences. I have takeaways from each relationship that helped me be a better person. I hope the others all did as well. Learning is something a person should want to do each day.

I never really wanted to kill myself, even though I came close a couple of times. I was at a few forks in the road and luckily, I took the right turns. One bad decision and I wouldn't be sitting here today writing. Deep down I just wanted to kill off the pain I was feeling at times. Plus, now I realize that no matter what goes wrong, or how much I dislike myself at times, there are people who love me. They are always better off with me living. I couldn't intentionally do that to the people that love me and would miss me.

At this point in my life right now, I'm over fifty. I want to live. I don't want to miss things. I'm afraid to miss out on future moments with my loved ones. I'm afraid of not being there for people when they need me. I want to watch everyone grow old and find themselves. I am not afraid of what will become of me after I die. Although I have faith in God, the unknown can be a frightening thought. It is inevitable and nobody can avoid it. I pray when the time comes, I am ready, and so are the people I leave behind. I pray that I don't take after my parents, because they both died young. Other than this bum back of mine, I feel young inside.

Despite the obstacles that were consistently put on my plate in life, I have fought every time I was challenged. I learned from my mistakes, and I tried to learn even more from the mistakes of others around me. I knew I had challenges early on as a skittish, stuttering kid who peed his pants because he was too afraid to talk to anyone. I envied the idea of being normal, or average. As time went on, I learned to mimic what others did around me, so I would appear to be.

I spent my life trying to find out what normal was. I found out that I had spent so many years trying to be what others expected me to be, I didn't even know who I was, or if I ever did before now. I have thrived to make today and tomorrow better than yesterday for years. I fail some days, but the next day I try again. As my dad taught me, "I will never give up". I will never give up on my dreams.

I still get depressed, but I try to remember that it's temporary. I know what makes me happy, so I surround myself with as much of that as possible. At the same time, I know what makes me sad or anxious, so I avoid those things as much as possible too. I also look bad on some bullets I have dodged especially when I was in my twenties. Jimmy didn't dodge those bullets. He spent his life as a drug addict felon, that all ended a few years back at age forty-two. I was about to reach out to him because I wanted him to meet Nathalia. He was cremated. It's still hard to imagine how they put that six-foot two man inside of a little box.

For myself, Self-awareness is the key to positive mental health. The older I become, the more I also realized that I have a lot to be happy for, and I understand that some days I won't always see it that way. Most people have some sort of struggle, in some way. I'm not the only one, yet it's hard to see that at times. Not much is what it appears to be on the surface. You need to dig deep down to find it. I found my self-worth, and realized that I needed to work on it, and I have. That will be a work in progress until the day I die. I will always try to learn from experiences and maintain being the best version of myself, even though I know that will look different every day.

I had spent most of my life craving love and attention and searching for a sense of purpose and security. It took damn near fifty years to calculate my thoughts and figure out who I really was. A huge piece of the puzzle was that I met Nathalia. Having a supportive, positive person by my side has been priceless in my healing and personal growth.

I love all my children very much; I believe that they are what kept me out of trouble all these years. They gave me purpose. Someone I had to face if I made a bad decision. Despite a few mistakes, I believe that I was a pretty good dad. Why? Because I sincerely cared and did my best... with what I had to work with. A lot of people can have kids, but being a good parent isn't easy, and like anything else in life it is a learned skill. I missed out on a lot with my two oldest and that is no one's fault. Life is just tricky like that.

I keep all my kids close to my heart, even though the relationships have been challenged at times. They are grown and have their own lives now. I don't always agree with the things that some do at times, same as most parents I suppose. I do accept what is and what I cannot change though. They know me, and they have always had a father present. I'm always here for solid, loving, non-biased advice.

I have never claimed to be perfect, but I have done a lot of good things too, even though I'm more than often judged only on mistakes. I wish that some situations throughout my life were handled better, but I sincerely gave it my best, whatever my best looked like at that time. I wasn't provided with many tools for success, and often what tools I gained were taken away, figuratively speaking. One of my greatest fears is failure. My willingness is one tool that only I have control of. I've kicked rocks a hundred times over, then always wiped away my tears and searched for a better way. I cannot truly fail unless I give up. Until then, I am getting one step closer to success with each failure, each lesson I learn and from every challenge I have yet still to face.

I learned to not sweat the small stuff, at least I always keep that mind set, even though some days are easier than others to achieve that. I try to only stress over the things I have control over, which isn't much anymore. I believe more now that everything that is meant to be, will be. I'm manifesting a better tomorrow and putting in the effort to make that happen. Being at peace with myself is what I thrive for each day.

I am engaged in my art and writing as I take life to the next phase. My latest works are extraordinary. Not because I think so, but that is what I have been told. I battle physical and emotional pain every day, but I now have the time, skill, and life experience to be the artist I was meant to be. The first part of my journey has ended, and the next part has begun.

Even though I have always been an artist, it didn't come first over the years. I will Never give up on it, no matter what bullshit gets thrown my way. Because an artist is who I am. It doesn't mean making money, it means being free to think, and create. Discovering my artistic style took a lifetime. I enjoy freely painting with an easel and a paintbrush, but my unique puzzle compositions are my invention, and they are extraordinary. I do believe that my brightest, shining moment is yet to come.

I taught myself to simply appreciate each day. I guess that happens naturally when ya get a little older. I try living each day like it's my last, with the mentality of knowing tomorrow will likely come. I know there are some people that have had it much worse than myself, but everything in life is relative and this was, and is, my life to live, and my thoughts to process. We walk down a path in life that veers in different directions every day. One bad choice and we end up on the wrong path trying to find the way back to the path intended. I am lucky to have veered back onto the right path as I went along. I pray that always continues.

I have absorbed a lot from life, and I've done a lot of learning the hard way. I got through tough times with perseverance. I can only do the best that I can sincerely do, after that it's in God's hands. The best one can do shouldn't mean sacrificing one's mental health doing it either. Even though life left me with some trauma, I don't regret any of it. Every experience in my life made me who I am today and will ultimately lead me to where I am supposed to go. I grew to learn that I am responsible for creating my own happiness. That task is easier for some than others, depending on the foundation life started on, the road traveled to get there, and willingness to learn.

I don't regret my path, even though it has been damaging. If I didn't make the choices I made, I may not have my children or my beautiful wife, Nathalia. I wouldn't have the wisdom to manage life. Everything up until now needed to happen. I needed to feel the pain before I could appreciate and understand life. Although, I've accepted that I won't always feel so optimistic every day, but not veering far off is key.

It took me half a century to realize that life will always be a challenge. It's like a game of chess. I need to think clearly before making moves. It's always important for me to learn from my own mistakes and the mistakes of others around me. I know that when I walk by the mirror, I won't always like who I see, but that's all I got. I am a strong person, but I've learned that I am emotionally vulnerable. I'm Blessed to be alive with my freedom, with loved ones around me.

The summer of twenty-two was an amazing summer. Nathalia and I had the summer off for different reasons, and the sun shined bright every single day, almost no rain at all. We went to Godard Park beach almost every day. A beach where my parents used to take me as a kid.

Right by the entrance of the beach is a restaurant, the same one my uncle owned when I was a little kid. We ate the best fried mozzarella I've ever tasted there. We walked the shore and collected the prettiest fan-like seashells. We smoked some weed in public because it was finally legalized. I enjoyed the peace. Sitting on our beach chairs that we set up under a beach umbrella, we began writing.

What I am is everything I've seen and everything I have experienced thus far. Eras in life came and left, it goes by fast. One thing I have always been, is an artist. Going back to sitting on the kitchen floor as a kid drawing pictures, to where I am today inventing new creations on canvas. I am a lover of beauty and harmony, searching through life's palette for the perfect colors to create the composition of my own life. An artist is what I will always be.

Even as I write the end of this book, things are happening and rapidly changing around me. Some things are great like my new kittens that we named Picasso and Dali, plus my youngest is having her first child, my fifth grandchild. Life is still moving forward each day throwing new curve balls, and challenges to overcome. That will never end. Life can be miserable, but it's those moments that we get to smile, or laugh if we are lucky, and that's what keeps us going strong. I've learned to embrace the good times, because I never doubt that a bad day will come. On those bad days I try to remember that it will pass, and I will smile again even though it doesn't seem that way in the moment. I'll wipe my tears and crack my half-smile because I know that better days are coming.

I'm not sure what will be written in the blank pages of my story that I have not been lived yet. For I am not dead, I am very much alive. The past is over, and the future is only in my imagination. What will I make it be, uncertain of how to end a story about a life that hasn't ended yet.

I never know when a moment is a moment to cherish until that moment has passed. So, I will Love strong and think clearly with an open mind, and an open heart. I will Live every day with my eyes wide open to not miss a moment I might one day cherish. Waking up this morning was a blessing, and until I no longer do, I will remember my father's words and never give up on chasing my dreams.

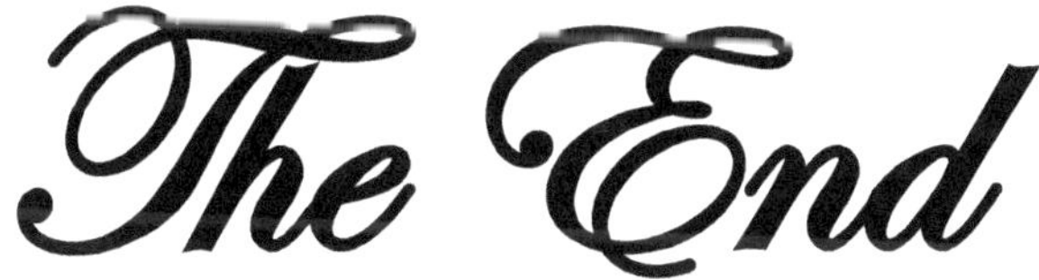

www.ingramcontent.com/pod-product-compliance
Lightning Source LLC
LaVergne TN
LVHW050511100826
845148LV00002B/299

* 9 7 9 8 8 9 4 4 3 8 6 0 3 *